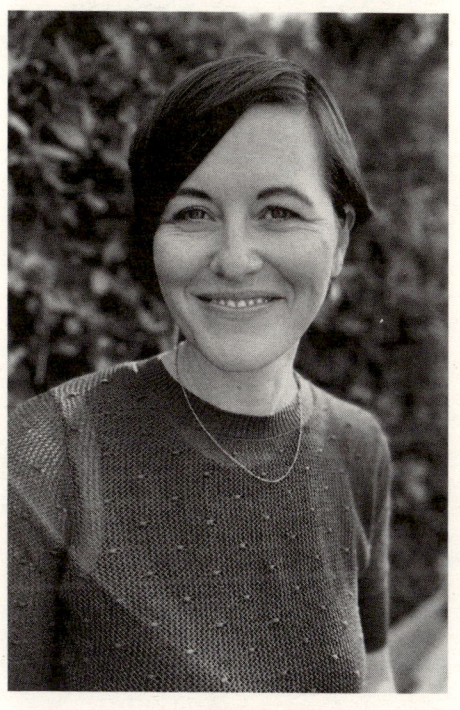

Bridget McNulty is a writer, diabetes advocate and co-founder of Sweet Life, South Africa's largest online diabetes community. She lives in Cape Town, South Africa, with her husband, son and daughter, and loves nothing more than a cup of tea and a good book – preferably somewhere green and leafy.

Find out more at www.bridgetmcnulty.com

DAILY GLIMMERS

The art of finding tiny joys
every day of the year

BRIDGET MCNULTY

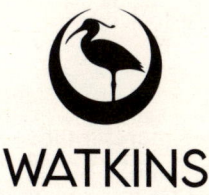

WATKINS

Daily Glimmers
Bridget McNulty

This edition first published in the UK and USA in 2025
by Watkins, an imprint of Watkins Media Limited
Unit 11, Shepperton House
89-93 Shepperton Road
London N1 3DF

enquiries@watkinspublishing.com

Commissioning Editor: Sophie Blackman
Managing Editor: Brittany Willis
Project Manager: Gigi St John
Illustrator: Lauren Fowler
Designer: Sneha Alexander
Head of Design: Karen Smith
Production: Uzma Taj

10 9 8 7 6 5 4 3 2 1

Printed and bound by CPI Group (UK) Ltd, Croydon, CR0 4YY

A CIP record for this book is available from
the British Library

ISBN: 978-1-78678-990-7 (Hardback)
ISBN: 978-1-78678-991-4 (eBook)

www.watkinspublishing.com

The manufacturer's authorised representative in the EU for product
safety is eucomply OÜ - Pärnu mnt 139b-14, 11317 Tallinn, Estonia,
hello@eucompliancepartner.com,www.eucompliancepartner.com

MIX
Paper | Supporting
responsible forestry
FSC® C013604

CONTENTS

Is it Autumn or Fall? Enter here!

Is it Winter? Enter here!

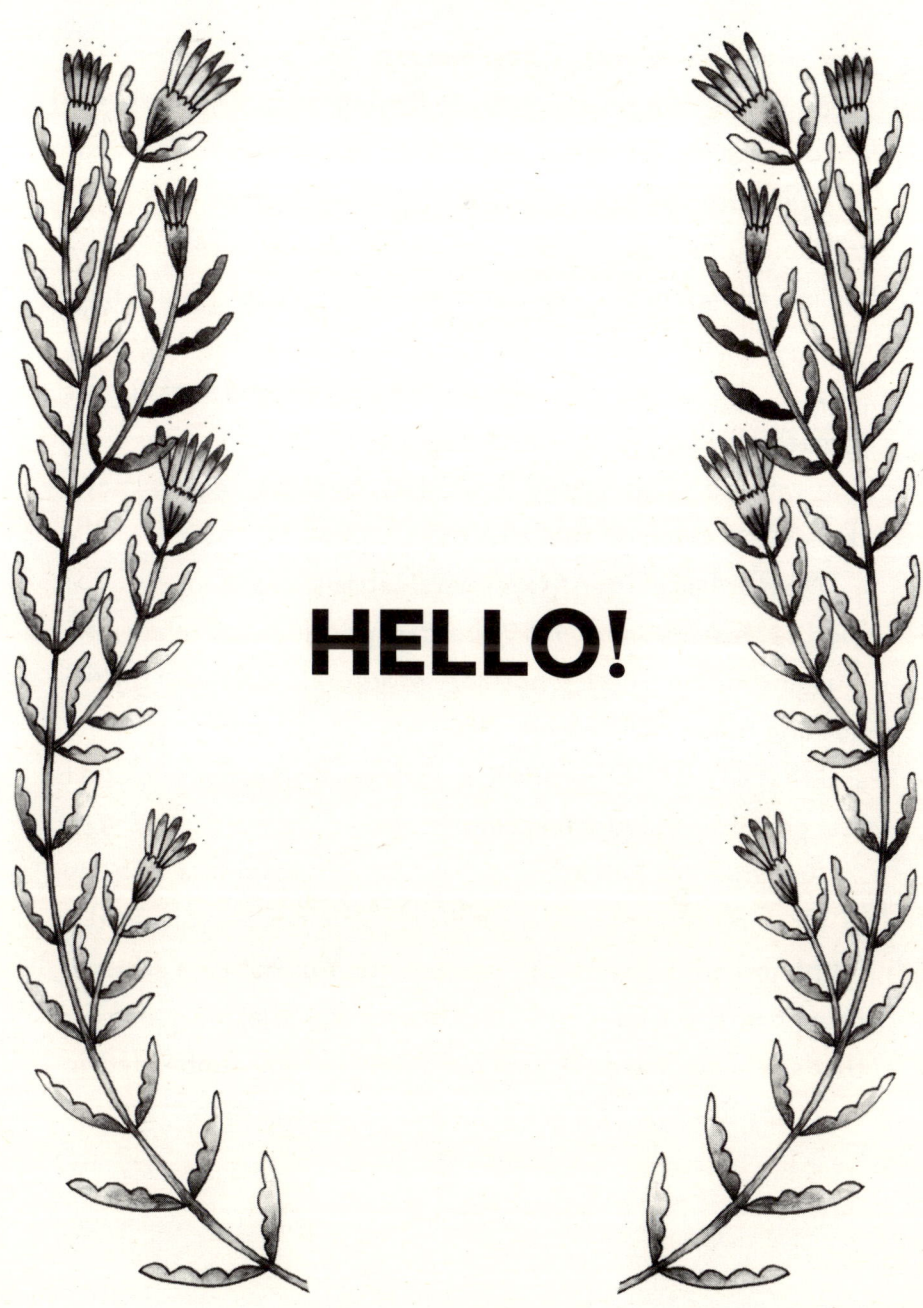

HELLO!

Welcome! I'm so happy you're here. You are in for such a treat. You're now on a journey to finding more glimmers, and uncovering more three-second slices of joy in your daily life.

The truth, as you know, is that life is often hard, and frequently boring. The drudgery of adult life is real: never-ending admin, near-constant overwhelm, a background hum of anxiety and a sense that you've got to keep it all together, or else. It can feel like you're clinging on and looking for something – anything – that might help. But not something that will add to your daily To Do List, because heaven knows there's too much on that already!

What's the solution? Glimmers. Little slices of joy.
Picture this: it's an ordinary Tuesday morning. You're at work, plugging away. There's nothing wrong, exactly, but there's nothing much right, either. You know you should be grateful and that so many others have it so much worse, but you don't feel grateful. You just feel kind of blah.

And then, at lunchtime, while you're sitting in a thin ray of sunshine eating an okay sandwich, you look at a tame little fountain and – there! Did you see it? You notice a rainbow caught in the spray, and your heart lifts. That's a glimmer: that's all you need. A small moment of joy embedded in everyday life.

WHAT ARE GLIMMERS?

The term "glimmers" was coined by clinician and author Deb Dana, who describes them as "micro-moments of regulation that foster feelings of wellbeing."[1] They are tiny noticings, specific to you, that make you smile. In other words: little slices of joy.

Glimmers are small fleeting moments that you notice. **Slices of joy** are chunkier and more likely to be crafted by you. They are both about seeing what is right in front of you (yet often easy to ignore). I use both terms interchangeably.

Therapist Helen Marie describes glimmers as tiny moments of awe.[2] There's that word tiny again, have you noticed? Doesn't it feel like a relief? You don't have to do anything big here: it's simply a few seconds of beauty. Here, and then gone. A moment of joy, a moment of calm, a brief sense of ease. And ease, in the midst of a busy, overwhelming, over-scheduled life, is a beautiful thing.

Joy spotting every day

Chade-Meng Tan, Google's former Happiness Guru, has a slightly-different-but-very-similar approach, which he calls "thin slices of joy": "Thin slices of joy occur in life everywhere … and once you start noticing it, something happens, you find it's always there."[3] The concept is simple: instead of waiting for The Next Big Thing to make you happy – a holiday, a life partner, a promotion, a child – you look out for three-second moments in your everyday life that lift your spirits.

HOW GLIMMERS WORK

Glimmers are micro-moments that can help your mood to shift and lift. Not dramatically: you're not being asked to "snap out of it". This is a soft approach: glimmers tell your nervous system that it's safe to calm down, and gently move you in the direction of physical and psychological wellbeing.

As Deb Dana explains, glimmers appear frequently in everyday life, and yet they go unnoticed. That's because your brain is wired to look for danger, and to pay more attention to negative events, trying to protect you. Luckily, you can change this wiring as you notice glimmers more and more and attune your nervous system to them. This noticing shifts things slightly. Life feels a little calmer, a little more hopeful.

Noticing glimmers is not about pretending that life is all sunshine and rainbows. "It's important to understand that glimmers are not a form of toxic positivity," explains Deb Dana. "They are not a way to always look on the bright side or count your blessings and discount your suffering." That is essential to me. I don't want to be peddled something that is emotionally inauthentic. Joy is a personal experience, unique to you. It might be merely a moment and – by its very nature – fleeting, but it's there.

It feels like the great equalizer because while everyone might not have access to Happiness with a capital H, you do have access to small moments when you think, "Oh, that's quite nice." And that's all you need. Quite nice.

HAPPINESS OR JOY?

So, why isn't this book about happiness?

Happiness is ...

caused by external factors. I'm happy when I'm given a present, a delicious meal, a fabulous holiday. It's a sparkly veneer laid over everyday life. It's not the most frequent visitor, I'm not going to lie. "I'm happy!" I'll say out loud when it arrives. "Good," my husband will respond.

I also find happiness in moments when the stars align and things are pleasantly ticking along. You're not worried about anyone, or anything, and just for a moment, you feel happy. It's a wonderful thing.

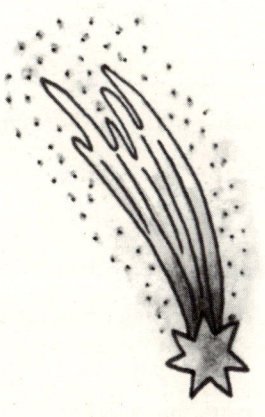

Happiness emerges as a lovely background when everything in life is peaceful. When everyone is healthy, when work is calm and productive, and

I don't have anything to worry about, I'm happy. It's like a shooting star – so beautiful! So fleeting. Happiness, to me, is dependent. If you're grieving, or stressed or depressed, forget about it. It's too far away and hard to grasp, too ephemeral.

Joy is ...

accessible in even the darkest moments, if you know how to look for it. It can't be taken from you, no matter what is going on in the rest of your life. It's an attitude and a practice. To look for joy is a daily choice. Given this exact life: right here, right now, what do you choose to focus on?

Joy is not simply a matter of eating your favourite snack every day and ticking joy off the To Do List. Sensory joy is impermanent, and you get used to it. That's why rich people stop noticing they're rich after a while, and just assume that everyone has a butler.

Joy is, by its very nature, not constant. It is a little glimmer or spark that you appreciate even as it starts dissipating. That's why I like the term glimmers: the idea of impermanence is baked into the name. Nothing brings you joy if you repeat it day in and day out, repeatedly, forever. But a chance encounter that brings a moment of delight can lift your day, regardless of what else is going on.

Joy feels manageable. It's like an underground stream, quietly burbling away, constantly available. There's less pressure to line everything up to achieve it – it can bubble up in the midst of heartbreak and stress, and doesn't require the stars to align. "Joy is moment to moment," Chade-Meng Tan explains, "the building block of happiness."

Yes, please.

FROM GRATITUDE TO GLIMMERS

While we're defining things, shall we take a quick look at gratitude? I have a few bones to pick with it ... For starters, gratitude is in the past. You write down what you're grateful for at the end of the day, rather than being mindful of what's happening as it's happening.

There's also a sense of pressure to be grateful even when things suck, because other people have it harder than you. I know that other people have it harder than me, almost all the time. But when I'm feeling down, that doesn't make me feel any better; it just makes me feel guilty. And that's a slippery waterslide to get on, because there is always (always) someone who is struggling more than you are, and before you know it you're dunked underwater with other people flailing about on top of you. There's no gratitude down there.

The Stoics (also mentioned on page 190) have an elegant way around this. Instead of guilting yourself into feeling grateful even when you don't, they suggest recognizing that you are living someone else's Dream Life. And then reflecting what it is about your very ordinary, seemingly unspectacular life that would make it someone else's Dream Life. A fridge full of food, four walls that don't let the wind in – that kind of thing. It's a surprisingly powerful exercise, and pretty much the only way I can make gratitude work for me.

Maybe gratitude, slices of joy and glimmers are interchangeable in your mind and if so, go right ahead calling them whatever works for you! If, on the other hand, you jumped on the gratitude bandwagon when it was rolling through town a few years ago and didn't dig the ride, I assure you slices of joy are a different experience.

This present moment

Glimmers and slices of joy are both about being present. Noticing this: right here, right now. Reading a book – awesome. Sitting somewhere comfortable, I'm guessing? Great. A few minutes to yourself: wonderful. And yes, other people don't have the luxury of sitting here reading a book, but this is not a gratitude competition. It's recognizing that in the midst of Everything That's Going On, this small moment is quite lovely.

Glimmers often reveal themselves when you give them time to unfurl. Joanna Gray, author of *The Little Book of Joy*, suggests The Five Minute Rule as an avenue to joy. If you leave the house five minutes earlier than you need to, it allows for a moment of peace or a surprise joyful encounter. I love that! Consciously building in time for glimmers to emerge.

I feel like the JOMO movement builds on this idea, too: the Joy Of Missing Out. Instead of squeezing happiness out of every moment, and filling your day with Fun Things, the idea is about choosing what you really want to do with your time – and only doing that. Uncovering the joy in your life according to your own rules, not as society dictates. And relishing all the things you're missing out on.

My glimmers journey

I've been on this joy journey for a long time – at least 25 years. I've been hunting for moments of sweet wildness and writing my version of gratitude journals (where I catalogue moments that feel wonderful amid days that do not), since I was a teenager.

There were some misguided steps on my joy journey, I admit. When I was 15, I had the delightful/annoying habit of gifting sweet little cards and pictures to people I knew – and also to total strangers. I would write down inspiring quotes and decorate them, and then slip them into unexpected places: under pillows, in postboxes and on the walls of elevators. The year I wore fairy wings, carried a wand and didn't wear shoes was adorable but perhaps a little odd for a 16-year-old. I decided my friends and I needed to visit sick people in hospital and give them cheery notes, and we found ourselves in the high-care ward, barefoot.

The nurses were, rightly, unimpressed.

Similarly, the amount of food colouring I put into everything I baked for several years was probably unhealthy – but bright pink cookies are so fun! Green banana bread is hilarious. Blue pancakes? Yes, please.

Glimmers have guided me on my joy journey. They offered me hope when I moved halfway across the world when I was 19. Hunting for slices of joy helped me through a type 1 diabetes diagnosis, when I was three days away from a coma and thought my life, as I knew it, was over. The concept was a lifeline during the first year of two kids (a newborn and a toddler and zero personal space ...). It helped me through my mom dying very suddenly and my dad having colon cancer, surgery, six months of chemo and a stroke. Grief hit me sideways and anything more than a few seconds of feeling okay seemed insurmountable.

Happiness? Excitement? Anticipation? Glee? Impossible. A few seconds of "Ah ... that's nice"? Possible. Joy when life is both awful and beautiful.

A healthy balance

And then there's the fine line between being grateful, noticing the beauty of life, and being insufferable. For example, I love an awe walk.[4] Going for a walk specifically to find awe-inducing things: that mountain view! The way that leaf has curled into itself! That stone the exact colour of sunset ... amazing! Some people are open to me pointing these things out, but I have learnt that if you want to have friends who will agree to go on walks with you, you don't exclaim over every single moment of beauty. It disrupts the conversation somewhat.

The whole point of finding slices of joy and noticing glimmers isn't so you can share them on social media (sorry). It's to gift yourself these small moments of delight that make your life feel better. That's it.

JOY DESPITE

What truly brought slices of joy alive for me was this edge of darkness they hint at. It's not joy through rose-tinted glasses, pretending that nothing bad is going on in the world. It's not ostriching yourself from reality, or cutting yourself off from people who are having a hard time. It's not judging yourself when you're struggling or when life is legitimately hard. It's joy despite. Despite the fact that things are going wrong all the time and everything is terrible. Or maybe because of it.

The truth is that although the world can be awful and terrible (and a quick glance at the news will confirm that it is awful and terrible in 1,001 different ways), it is also hopeful and beautiful. Humans are making unthinkable, unfathomable decisions every day. And yet, humans are also wonderful, kind and generous. There are tiny glimmers, despite it all.

Glimmers are fleeting and impermanent, and it's hard to know when they will visit or when they will leave. But isn't that a metaphor for life? You are gifted this one life, and you don't know how long it will be, but you have this day, today. By treasuring each experience as a maybe-last-time, you're more able to appreciate it. By recognizing that your life is not endless, you can see the beauty in the small things.

And that's really what this book is about. If there's one thing I have learnt how to do – through diabetes, grief, work and parenting – it's to find the lightness in the everyday. No matter how ordinary and dull you might think your life is, it is peppered with these jewels of pleasure and joy, just waiting to be noticed.

GLIMMERS CAN CHANGE YOUR LIFE

Hunting for glimmers and slices of joy is the most low admin way to improve your life. They don't cost anything or add anything to your To Do List. You're probably experiencing them already without noticing. Did you just take a sip of tea and think, "Mmm …"? That's a slice of joy. Get a sweet message from a friend? There's another. Stretch and feel your muscles release? Lovely!

Because they're so brief and fleeting, these small moments are easy to miss – they're the kind of thing that pass by unnoticed unless you're really looking for them. Finding and noticing glimmers – on the commute to work or while doing daily tasks – is an art, a skill and a practice. Looking for glimmers isn't a distraction from life; it's a coping method. It's a mental health practice to enable you to deal with the darkest days.

This book outlines how to notice glimmers, and why it's so important for your wellbeing. It's a practical, useful way to start feeling better about your life, no matter what it looks like right now.

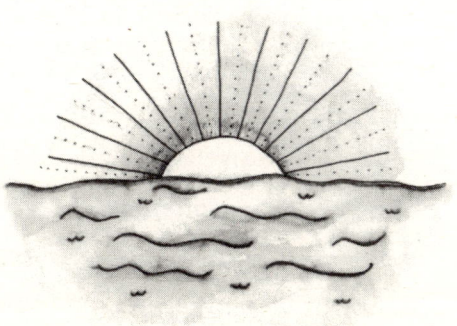

Life is often hard, and happiness can be elusive. Joy, though, is accessible in even the darkest moments, if you know how to look for it. Let's look for it, together. Every day.

HOW TO FIND GLIMMERS EVERY DAY

I know that it can be hard to access an appetite for joy sometimes. Real Life can be so drudgy and filled with washing up to do, appointments to make and tasks to complete that it can be difficult to know where to even start looking for glimmers. That's why the goal here is: one glimmer a day. One three-second moment where you think, "Ah ... that's nice." You're not aiming for marvellous or wonderful or fantastic ... simply nice.

365 slices of joy

Every day, I've given you an idea for a slice of joy you might be able to find. And then a couple of other, aligned, suggestions in case that one doesn't resonate with you. Feel free to ignore the ones you don't like, or create your own private collection of glimmers you chanced upon because you were on the lookout. It is remarkable how much you notice when your eyes are trained on a specific topic.

I've tried to make the slices of joy as evergreen as possible, but some of them will be hard Noes for you, perhaps unrelatable, or not your kind of joy-sparking activity. I am a straight white woman living on the tip of Africa. I have two young children and love spending time alone, and could eat fruit and chocolate all day. I have a very specific lens that I'm looking at the world through, and the glimmers in this book are the things that bring me joy, as I look through that lens. I've tried, as much as possible, not to make the slices of joy exclusionary. I'm allergic to cats, but when I asked my #slicesofjoy community, they gave me an abundance of cat-specific glimmers, so I had to include them. Dogs, too.

Seasons and themes

The book is organized by seasons and themes, so that you can explore the many ways glimmers appear in your life. The world has so many sensory delights to offer up, if you can pay attention to their whispers.

I'll also share with you some of the wisdom I've collected on the subject of joy, like colourful marbles I've been carrying around in my pockets – helpful ways to uncover more joy in your daily life, reflections on the long history of slices of joy, the science behind it and a few personal anecdotes and confessions.

Where to begin? Today! Whatever day that is for you. You could turn to the page for the season you're in so that the glimmers suit your life right now. Or turn to a theme that speaks to you. If you want to dip in and out of this book for a year, go right ahead. If you want to read it all in one day, please do.

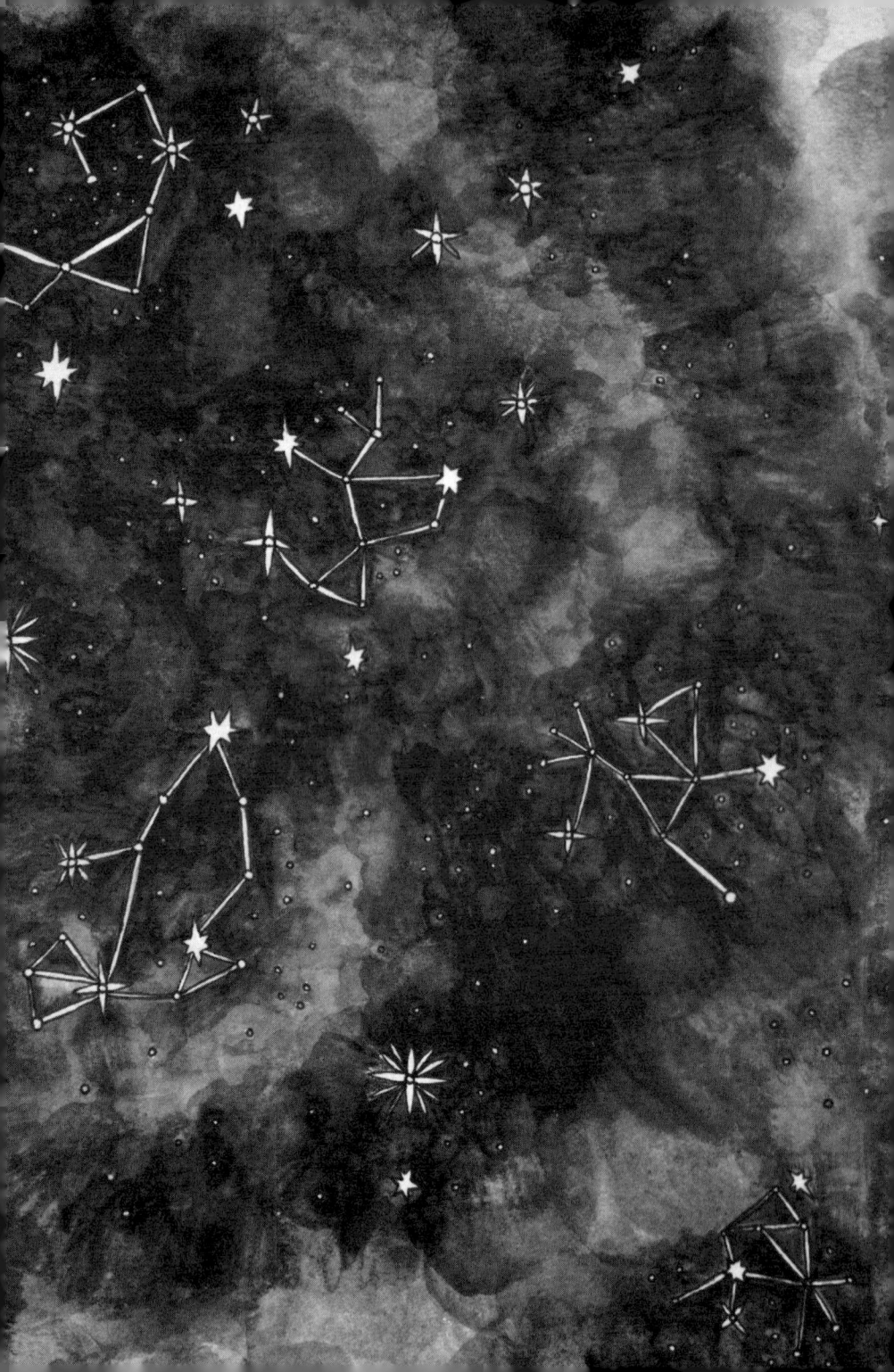

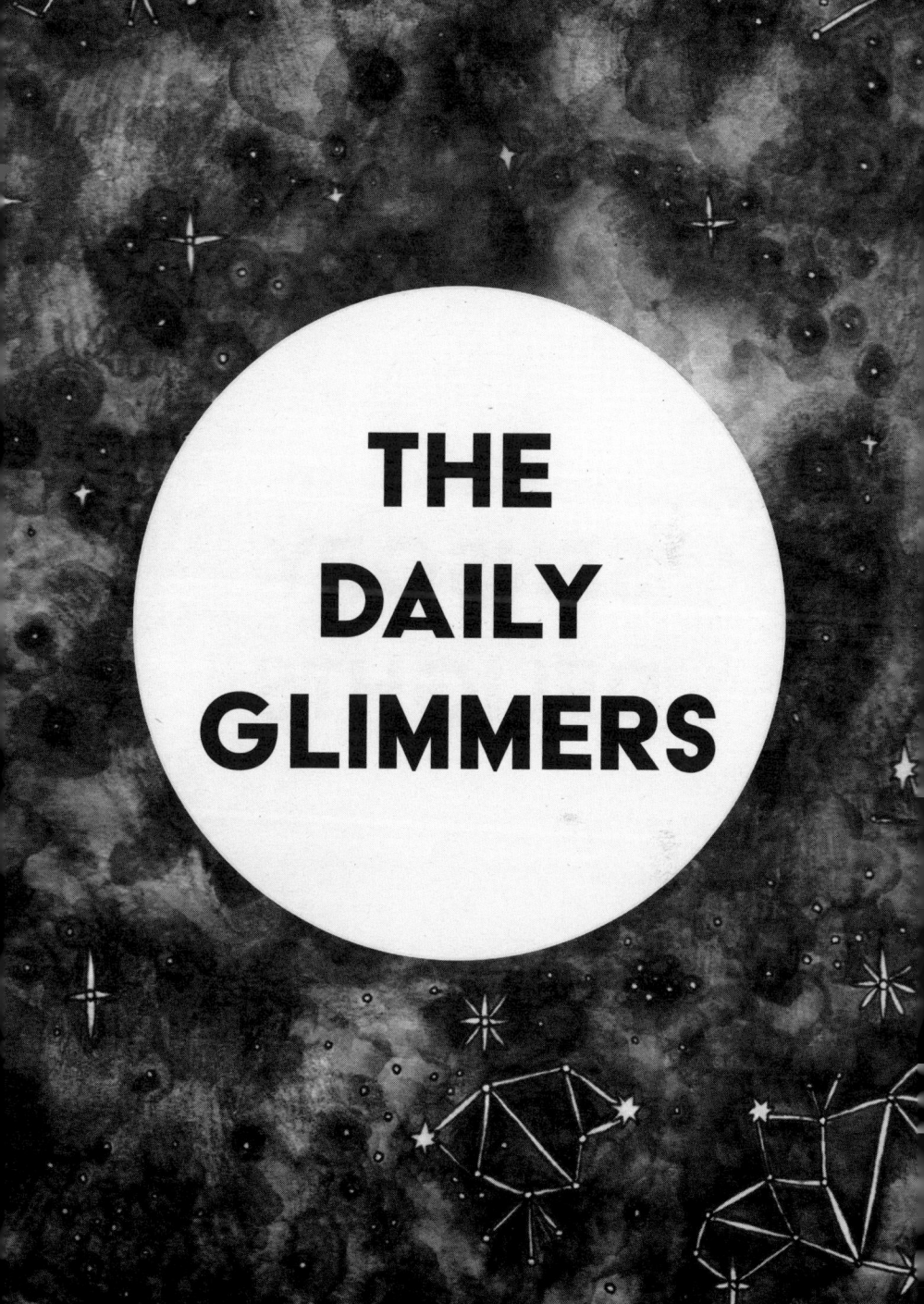

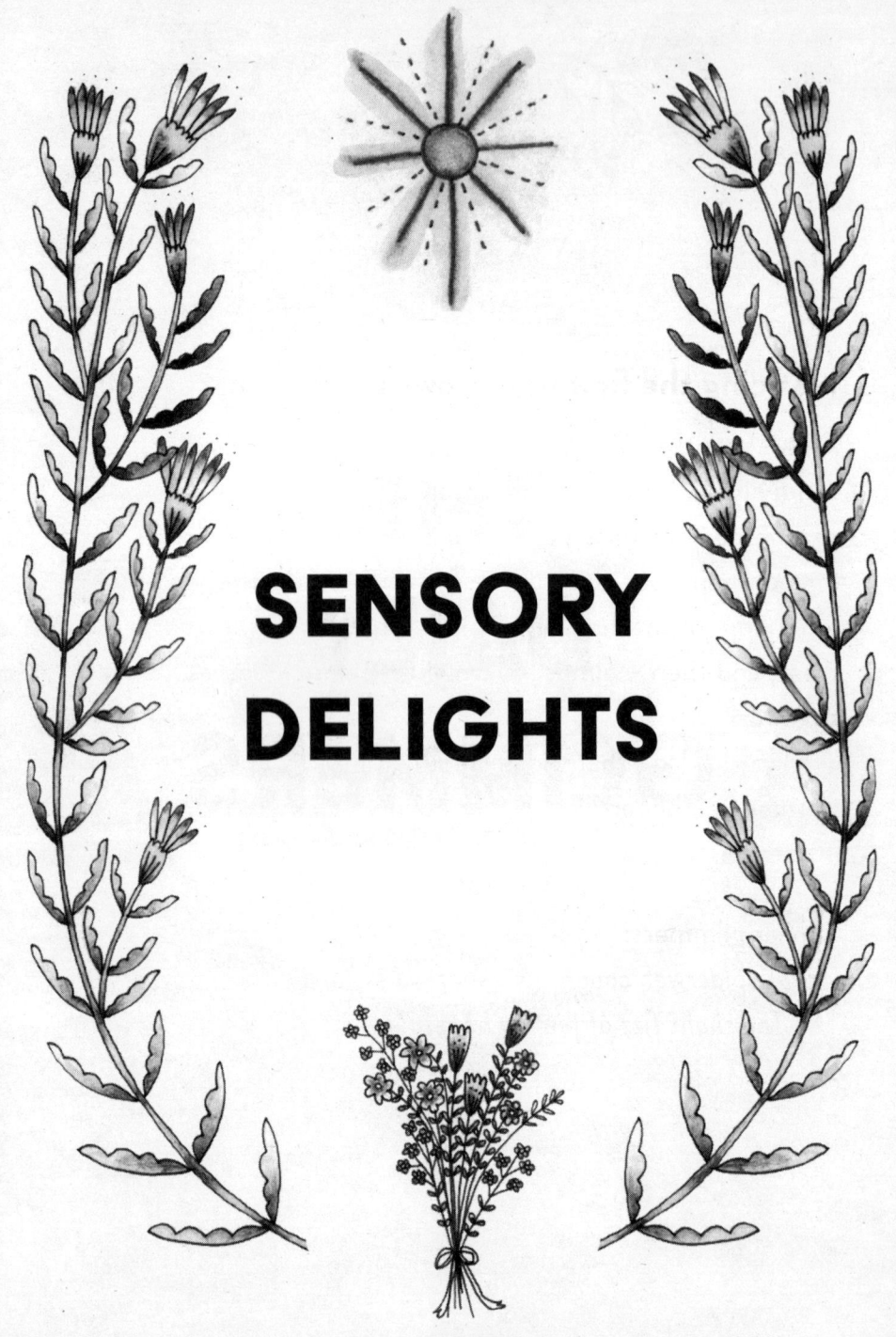

SENSORY DELIGHTS

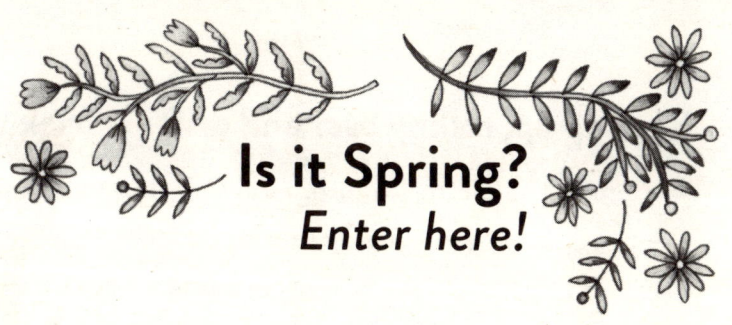

Is it Spring?
Enter here!

Noticing the first new growth of the year

After months of cold and grey and hard and brown, suddenly! A little shoot of green ... That first spring growth can be easy to miss because it's so slight and delicate, but if you keep your eyes peeled you'll see small green things emerging from the earth, and buds starting to form on trees, and then – almost overnight it seems – leaves starting to unfurl.

Unfurl ... Isn't that the perfect word for what you do when warmer weather arrives? Shuck off your heavy coat and unfurl into the light.

Similar glimmers:
+ *A spiderweb caught in a shaft of sunlight.*
+ *The slight fizz of feeling hopeful.*

Waking up, rolling over and drifting back to sleep

For once, the alarm isn't on. And you don't wake up earlier than your body wants to. You swim up from a pleasant dream into wakefulness, then realize you don't have to get up yet (miracle of miracles!) Roll over to the other side, close your eyes and drift back asleep ... It's like someone pulling you into a warm hug. Simply marvellous.

Similar glimmers:
+ *The other side of the pillow.*
+ *Pulling a soft blanket up to your chin.*

Tiny self-seeded plants

There are few things in life that seem as miraculous to me as a tiny self-seeded plant. A gentle stalk and budding leaves growing out of the pavement, a teeny lavender that's been blown on the wind and taken root or a new miniature succulent emerging where a piece was broken off the original (my personal favourite). The miracle of plants forging ahead and creating new life is so hopeful, and such a testament to resilience.

Similar glimmers:
+ *The wind whispering through leaves.*
+ *Opening the windows wide to let in fresh spring air.*

Being given something homemade

My love language is gifts, so being given anything delights me. But being given something homemade or homegrown is so special. The time and love that was invested into it, the fact that someone was thinking of you while they made or gathered it, the rarity of the gift ... It all adds to the wonder.

Similar glimmers:
+ *A cutting from a friend's garden.*
+ *A child's drawing on the fridge – no matter what it looks like.*

The sound of the sea

The sound of waves lapping against the shore is so soothing because the rhythmic nature has a low frequency, which activates the parasympathetic nervous system, helping you to relax and unwind.[5] That's why spending time by the ocean can be so relaxing. Who knew?!

If you're not anywhere near an ocean, you can listen to recordings of ocean sounds while you're working, reading or to help you get to sleep ...

Similar glimmers:
+ *The gentle burble of a stream.*
+ *The delicate splash of a fountain.*

A bunch of fresh flowers

They can be a cheap-and-cheerful bunch from the store, a few handpicked blooms from the garden (weeds? who cares!) or a fancy bouquet. The arrangement doesn't matter: what matters is that they are fresh and beautiful. Flowers don't need to be productive or useful, except as a means to brighten your room and lift your mood for a moment.

Similar glimmers:
+ *Colouring in (anything, even just a doodle).*
+ *Writing with a lovely pen.*

A blank sheet of paper

Even if all you're doing is writing a shopping list, a fresh sheet of paper is so promising. The satisfaction of the pen scratching away, something emerging – words, pictures, shapes, doodles.

Similar glimmers:
+ *That new book smell.*
+ *The first page of a new journal. A whole book filled with potential (although sometimes I find the first page too intimidating to write on, so will just draw a star and turn the page!).*

The pitter-patter of raindrops

Rain falling outside is the definition of cosy, especially if you don't have to leave the house any time soon and can luxuriate in being warm and dry when outside it's cold and wet. If you can wrap your hands around a mug of something warm to drink and watch raindrops skitter across the windowpane, that's about as good as it gets. Even better if you're tucked up in bed, or if there's a crackling fire nearby.

Similar glimmers:
+ *Closing your eyes and listening to birds singing and bees humming.*
+ *A freshly wood-chipped flower bed.*

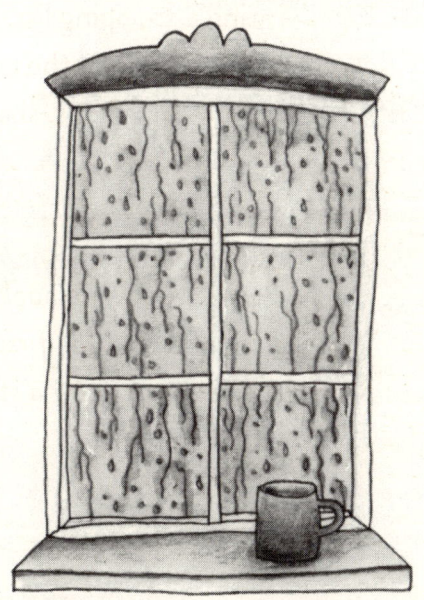

The first days of warmth

Does it feel a little warmer today? The days seem to be starting earlier, don't they? And lingering longer? At first, nobody wants to claim it for fear of being too hasty, but once you get one nice day followed by another ("nice" is relative, depending on what the winter has been like), there's a kind of softening into the fact that yes, this is *actually* spring. What a relief.

Similar glimmers:
+ *The almost universal lifting of spirits (and of eyes to meet other people's faces) when the weather improves.*
+ *That hopeful feeling when you have a good night's sleep after a long spell of bad nights.*

Driving through a big muddy puddle

Whether you're in a car or a bus, the "sploosh" of driving through a big muddy puddle and watching the spray arc up without making you wet is so deeply satisfying. Yes, please. More of these moments.

Similar glimmers:
+ *Driving in a heated car on a rainy day.*
+ *Bare feet stepping out onto dewy grass.*

Watering plants first thing in the morning

It could be a garden or a few potted plants on a ledge. Either way, there is something so right with a world (and a day) that begins with watering plants. It's an act of service that serves pleasure, a gift to the earth that gifts back a few moments of calm. A fulfilling of a need that is simple and satisfying.

Similar glimmers:
+ *A gentle breeze on a warm day.*
+ *The way a new coat of paint transforms a wall or piece of furniture.*

A back scratch

What is it about a back scratch that feels so heavenly? Is it because it's such an act of service? Because it's impossible to give yourself a back scratch, so it's precious when you receive one? Or is it the unmistakable relief of an itch being scratched? Whatever the reason, back scratches remain one of my all-time favourite slices of joy.

Similar glimmers:
+ *Exfoliating. Your skin feels rough, you rub on the exfoliator (or pull out the loofah) and a few minutes later your skin is soft and smooth. Ta-da!*
+ *Putting lip balm on dry lips.*

Magical salt

You know salt? That tasty but fairly boring stuff you put on your food? Well, a friend gave me some magical salt and I kid you not, it has transformed my taste-buds. Everything you put this salt on tastes more like itself. Tomatoes taste more like tomatoes (juicy, sweet, tangy). Cucumber tastes more like cucumber (crisp, green, fresh). Don't even get me started on buffalo mozzarella!

What I love even more than the salt itself (if that's possible) is how easy it is to make: mix pink Himalayan salt with dried olives, ground garlic and dried rosemary. Whizz it all up together and the end result is so much greater than the sum of its parts ... Truly, it's magical.

Similar glimmers:
+ *Tasting something new (and loving it!).*
+ *A mid-afternoon snack, right when you're feeling snackish.*

A city at night

Rooftops, buildings, windows, sparkling lights ... any city, town or village from a distance will do. I think it's something to do with the allure of distance. Up close, it's just street lights, fast food joints and stores that have shut for the day, but get some distance – a little perspective – and it all turns twinkly. Coordinated. Beautiful. All you have to do is step back and *look*.

Similar glimmers:
+ *Sequins catching the light and making rainbows.*
+ *Light slanting through the leaves of a tree.*

Classical music while you cook

A friend once suggested starting the weekend by playing classical music, because it somehow seems to stretch out Saturday morning and cast a peaceful sheen over the whole weekend. I love this idea! I've found it works really well for a weeknight dinner, too. It doesn't have to be classical music; it can be anything that you find soothing. The idea is simply to ground yourself in the present moment: right here, right now.

Similar glimmers:
+ *Turning the music up loud.*
+ *Chopping your way through a mound of vegetables.*

Sunshine pouring onto your back like honey

There is a particular flavour of sunshine that feels like a miraculous gift from the heavens. The kind that pours down, even if it's only for half an hour, and is so warm you can almost see the golden rays of vitamin D, and almost smell the honey-like scent.

It is particularly effective in contrast. When it's been a long, cold winter, that first spring warmth is one of the most tangible slices of joy you can feel. There it is, slanting out of a cloud, when you've just stepped out of a cold room. Savour that moment of delicious bone-tingling warmth.

Similar glimmers:
+ *Sunshine on your back after a cold swim.*
+ *An ice cream cone, preferably eaten in a ray of sunshine.*

Your first sip of tea or coffee for the day

There is something so delicious about the first sip of tea or coffee for the day. It's an invitation to your body to wake up, slowly begin the day and engage your mind in what might come next.

Similar glimmers:
+ *The aroma from a newly opened bag of coffee.*
+ *Early morning stillness when the air smells green.*

Everything in its right place

The books are all lined up. The kitchen containers have all found their lids. Clothes have been tidied away from the backs of chairs, and crumbs have been cleaned off counters. There is a brief moment when all is in order, and peace reigns. It does not – and cannot – last, but that doesn't take away from its brief beauty.

Similar glimmers:
+ *Sorting art supplies into colours.*
+ *The satisfaction of a beautifully tended patch of garden.*

Birds cooing when they think nobody is listening

Perhaps birds coo regardless of whether anyone is listening or not, but feeling like you're overhearing a private bird conversation is precious. It's a gentle, restful sound, wired to relax the brain. Scientific studies have shown that natural sounds affect the bodily systems that control the fight-or-flight and rest-digest autonomic nervous systems, so it's worth hunting for the natural sounds that deeply relax you.[6]

Similar glimmers:
+ *Gentle wind chimes (emphasis on gentle).*
+ *A solo nature walk, listening to all the sounds, smelling all the green.*

A softly scented candle

A good scented candle is a wonderful thing. It can suffuse the air with a soft scent that makes your shoulders drop and the corners of your mouth lift without you even noticing it. Some people dislike scented candles, and I am 100 per cent with them when it comes to aromas I don't like (vanilla, strawberry, anything fake). But there's a scent for everyone, I'm sure ... Give it a try (just make sure you sniff deeply before buying the candle so you know what you're in for!)

Similar glimmers:
+ *A pet-warmed bed.*
+ *Beautifully scented hand cream.*

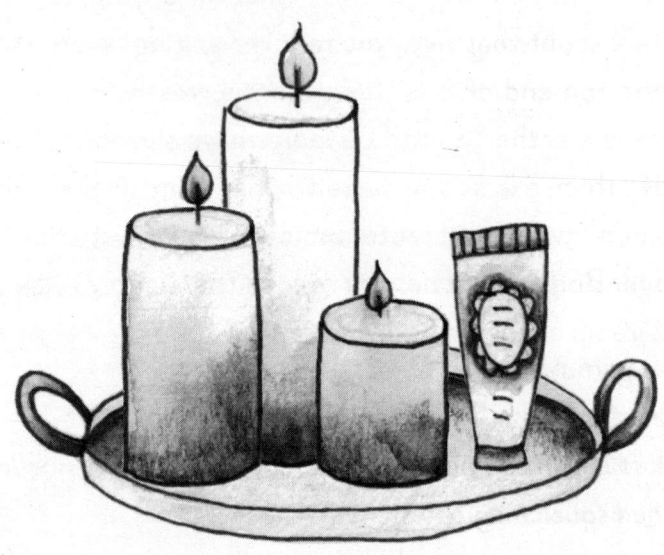

Taking a deep breath of sun-warmed flowers

"Stop to smell the roses" is pretty much the most twee advice anyone could offer. And yet, it is surprising how lovely sun-warmed flowers smell. Surprising, perhaps, because it's a rare moment that you're outside, in the company of flowers, and able to inhale them deeply. It doesn't have to be roses, naturally. Any flowers will do.

Similar glimmers:
+ *The way the scent of jasmine fills the evening air.*
+ *Laying a hand against a tree trunk and actually noticing the tree. It was there all along! But somehow easy to miss.*

Lush grass between your toes

Let's talk about toes for a second. They have such a hard job, stuck on the end of feet, being squashed into shoes all day. Once the weather warms up enough to set them free, can you give them a little wiggle and let them appreciate life for a moment or two? Fresh grass between your toes is like a mini massage. Bonus points if you're able to lie back on the grass and stare up at the sky while your toes have their moment.

Similar glimmers:
+ *Soft beach sand under bare feet.*
+ *Mud squelching between your toes.*

Clean sheets

David Sedaris, the American humorist, writes about changing his sheets three times a week so he feels like he's sleeping in a hotel.[7] While this is not an approach I can recommend (for environmental reasons, if nothing else), I do think he's onto something by caring so much about his bedding.

Clean sheets feel like a bedtime treat. The fresh scent, the crisp feeling – it's a little gift to yourself from yourself. Feeling down? Change your sheets! Future You will be so pleased at bedtime.

Similar glimmers:
+ *Something soft to wear to sleep in.*
+ *Freshly shaved legs slipping into a freshly made bed.*

The smell of dinner cooking

It's been a long day. You're pretty tired, pretty hungry and a little weary, to be honest. And then you smell dinner cooking, and it all melts away. The promise of a delicious meal, some downtime, a moment to press pause ... Thank heavens.

Similar glimmers:
+ *The waft of cake-scented air when you take a tray of cupcakes out of the oven.*
+ *The scent of fresh rosemary: a little spicy, a little surprising.*

Washing off the sticky smell after a night out

Jerry Seinfeld has a whole routine about how the purpose of going out is so that you can return home again. There is a real beauty in coming home after a night out and washing off that sticky or smoky smell before climbing into bed. It's the book-end to a successful evening, or the reward for getting through it (depending how the night went!).

Similar glimmers:
+ *Making a late-night hot drink when the house is quiet.*
+ *A debrief with friends after a particularly fun night out.*

Sliding your tongue across just-cleaned teeth

There is such pleasure in just-cleaned teeth after a dentist visit, isn't there? Not only in the sensation, but in knowing that something has been ticked off your list for another few months. You're winning at adulting! Well done you. Even everyday teeth cleaning can make you feel better – such an easy win!

Similar glimmers:
+ *Removing a face mask and feeling your baby-soft skin underneath.*
+ *Patting down wet sand to make it smooth.*

Putting on a pair of new socks

Songs should be written about That New Sock Feeling. The satisfaction of pulling up the socks and having them stay exactly where they should be. The softness of the sock itself. The freshness of knowing they've never been worn. The happy feeling they give your feet, toes wiggling merrily inside their new home. It doesn't last, of course, but perhaps that's part of the pleasure, knowing that it's fleeting ...

Similar glimmers:
+ *Freshly shaved cheeks.*
+ *Cosy slippers. More specifically, that moment you slip your feet inside them.*

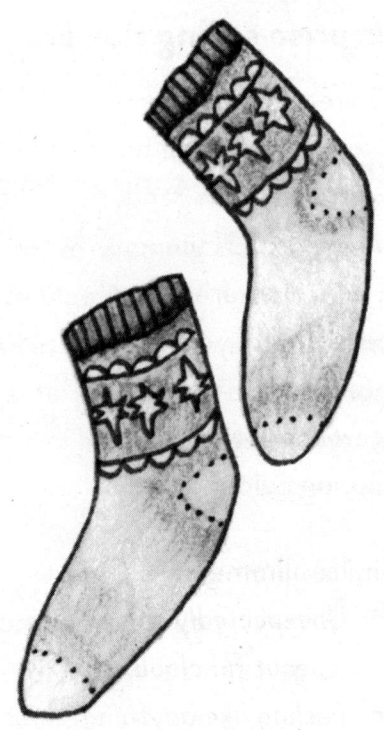

Cool cement floors

Bare feet on a cool cement or tiled floor. A pool of dark shade on a veranda where you can sit, your back against the outside wall. Often accompanied by a sense of relief and ease.

Similar glimmers:
+ *Cold water to drink mid-hike.*
+ *Walking across a thick carpet or sheepskin rug.*

Surprise spring flowers

Where do they come from? Who planted them? It is borderline magical how spring flowers pop up, in abundance, everywhere: on random roadsides and pavements, in parks and fields. Of course, there's also great delight in spring flowers that are lovingly planted in city flower beds, or that you planted yourself before the winter set in. I think it's because they carry with them the scent of possibility ... If, in a few short weeks, that unrelenting hard soil could produce amazing colour like that, well! What might *you* do today?

Similar glimmers:
+ *Unexpectedly spotting shapes: a heart-shaped rock or a beautiful cloud.*
+ *Feeling like anything is possible.*

Stepping out of a building into air that's the perfect temperature

There are probably – what? – four days a year when this happens? But every so often you'll step out of a building, perhaps from work, into fresh air that is somehow exactly the right temperature. There's no hint of "brr" or "phew", it's just right. Goldilocks weather.

In fact, it's sometimes so "just right" that it's hard to notice it: the absence of discomfort. But it's a sweet and beautiful thing to feel, even just for a few seconds.

Similar glimmers:
+ *Stepping indoors after being in the sun for hours.*
+ *The perfect temperature water as you step into the bath, sea or swimming pool.*

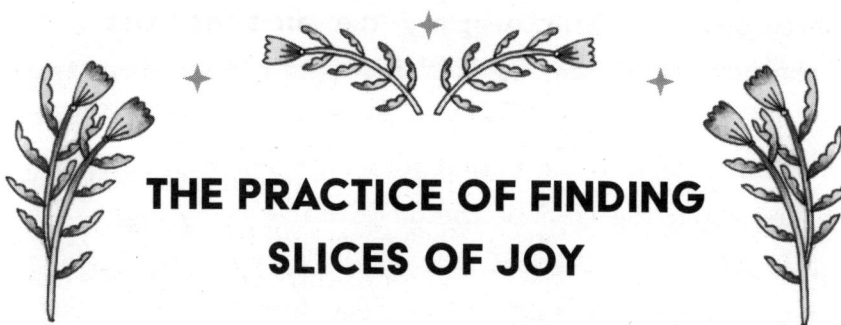

THE PRACTICE OF FINDING SLICES OF JOY

Finding slices of joy and noticing glimmers is a practice and – like any practice – not always easy. That's why it's called a practice, I suppose, because you have to keep working on it.

I won't lie, I thought I had this stuff down. I thought I had #slicesofjoy in my back pocket. But it turns out I need reminding, too. Realigning myself to the practice of finding slices of joy and training my eyes and my heart to notice glimmers is a consistent theme for me. Here's how I keep working on it.

✦ The lure of The Next Big Thing

It's very easy to make life about waiting for The Next Big Thing. I'm sure I'm not alone in this. The big holiday, the weekend away, the new purchase, the party ... all those things you think will make you happy.

The lure of The Next Big Thing is delicious: both the waiting, and the thing itself. Let me give you an example. A little while ago, we booked flights to the USA, to see three of my favourite people in the world and meet their babies. It was to be my kids' first international trip: two weeks of pure joy, a chance to reconnect with friends and celebrate life, love and all that good stuff. For six months, we talked about the USA at the dinner table every night. The anticipation was so sweet that it felt like we were breaking off tiny chunks of chocolate every day: from a bar that never seemed to end.

And then we went on the trip, and it was glorious! Hot, sunny and blue-skied, filled with friends and hugs and fun, ice cream and laughter and glee. We went to a carnival on a hot summer's night, marvelled at Fourth of July fireworks, swam in lakes and sailed around Boston Harbour on a pirate ship as the sun set. Truly, you couldn't make this stuff up.

And then we came home. A 5-hour train trip; a 15-hour flight. Home to a freezing cold house in midwinter. It was dark, cold and rainy. You know that back-to-earth feeling after a wonderful trip? The post-holiday blues at full volume.

I searched, somewhat frantically, for something to look forward to. We had a weekend getaway planned. My son's birthday. We could save for another holiday the following year. I mentally scrolled through all the options I could think of, and nothing worked.

So, I reached for gratitude: I have such a lovely home. My own bed is so much more comfortable than any of the beds we slept in on holiday. My family is healthy. I enjoy my work. But I couldn't grasp it. It all felt … flat. I sank into a funk.

This is my problem with gratitude. When you're already feeling low, asking yourself to appreciate what you have is too big an ask. Grief is the most stark example of this, because you can barely lift your head each morning, never mind greet it with gratitude. But a mild depression or even a case of the blues puts gratitude out of reach as well, in my experience. And then you beat yourself up for not appreciating what you have when so many other people have less … And nobody ever felt better after a bout of self-flagellation.

✦ The tiniest spark of light

The reality is that big trips, dream jobs and exciting adventures aren't the norm. That's not how life works. If you're constantly waiting for something exciting, much of life will be spent in a holding pattern, wishing the days away. Isn't that a waste?

It's when you're generally feeling blah about life that slices of joy really count. That's when you need to notice glimmers. I started small: only looking for three things a day, and giving myself a break once I'd found those. I suppose it was a gratitude journal, of sorts, except that instead of reflecting back at the end of the day, I consciously noticed the slices of joy as they were happening. I was on the lookout for the tiniest glimmer that might lift my spirits for a moment.

For example, our hot water had been acting up, leading to lukewarm showers on cold mornings. The first morning I had a hot shower on a cold day, I thought, "Ahhhh! Here it is: this is a slice of joy."

I had fallen out of the habit of exercising, and the first day I went for a walk on the mountain, it was tough. I was slow, my legs felt heavy, I really wasn't that into it. But then I got to the top of the hill and looked back at the view and thought, "Yes. This is a slice of joy."

What I love about this approach is the total absence of pressure. Things don't have to be big or impressive – in fact, almost by definition they are not. Glimmers are moments that pass fleetingly. You don't have to do anything to create them; all you have to do is notice them as they flit past.

Slices of joy have slightly more intention behind them in that you hunt them out, but the hunting can be as easy as reaching for a glass of water. Chade-Meng Tan says, "Right now, I'm a little thirsty, so I will drink a bit of water. And when I do that, I experience a thin slice of joy both in space and time. It's not like 'Yay!' It's like, 'Oh, it's kind of nice.'" I can do kind of nice. You can do kind of nice too, I'm sure.

✦ One good thing a day

My family has started a new ritual at dinner time where we each say one good thing that happened that day. Not the best, not our favourite, merely one good thing. My son said to me yesterday, "What if nothing particularly good happened? What if it was just A Day?"

And I explained to him that, on days like that, we look for the smallest things. A juicy bite of nectarine. Colouring in a picture. A really good hug. Swinging on a swing. We look for a tiny glimmer, no matter how small it might be.

These glimmers don't have to be frequent. You only have to notice a few of them throughout your day (even one will do!). There's no pressure to be in a constant state of joy.

✦ A low bar for delight

I'm actively working to lower my standards for joy. Like, what is the smallest possible thing that could lift my spirits for a moment ... This bite of sandwich? The sound of birds singing outside? A funny meme my friend just sent me? Any of those will do! It really doesn't need to be a Big Thing.

I'm aiming for a "low bar for delight", as writer Shauna Niequist recommends: "One of my goals is to be a person who is easily delighted, who can find great cause for celebration in a fig or a familiar face. If you need fireworks and perfection in order to crack a smile, you're going to be disappointed over and over when life fails to be spectacular on command."[8]

Every Small Thing counts. Tiny glimmers are the glue that hold life together. I don't think a happy life is composed of nonstop rainbows and cupcakes, one after another in a giddy technicolour explosion. I think it's more like a string of beads with enough shiny glimmers to add colour and light to every day.

✦ Priming your attention

One of the greatest gifts of joy spotting is that it primes your attention to see more lovely things. Your senses become attuned to noticing glimmers. They've always been there: this is nothing new. It's simply priming your attention in a certain direction. Priming is a psychological concept that explains how exposure to a certain stimulus makes you predisposed to noticing a subsequent stimulus, without a conscious connection. Have you noticed how when you're considering buying something (a new red top, for example), you notice them everywhere? This is the same idea. Imagine feeling hopeful about the fact that something tiny and delightful is going to happen to you today, and then noticing tiny and delightful things all day ... How fun! Put simply: the more you notice glimmers, the more you'll notice glimmers.

✦ A dedicated practice

This practice requires a certain amount of dedication. While writing this book, I diligently wrote down three tiny slices of joy a day, so that I could accumulate the ideas you see here. But then I reached the end of the notebook and I stopped. And guess what happened? I stopped noticing as many glimmers.

As soon as I realized this, I bought a new notebook and started my daily practice again (yes, it is that easy). I think it's more than the notebook being an accountability partner, though. I had given myself permission and – more importantly – made space for joy. Finding small moments of delight was a priority, and then it wasn't. And when things aren't a priority, I tend to let them slip. Making this a daily practice is essential. Ideally, pair it with something you do every day — read the daily glimmer as you sip your morning cuppa, or while you brush your teeth. "Habit pairing" is an enormously effective behavioural change tool, and will help you learn the habit of noticing glimmers.

✦ Slices of joy as a coping mechanism

Sometimes in life, finding slices of joy becomes an absolute necessity. The week before Christmas 2023, my dad had a severe stroke. All my worst fears about an elderly parent living alone came to life: he was lying on the floor for 15 hours before he was found. It was one of those days that are so awful you almost have to detach from reality to cope.

In the days and weeks that followed, I made a conscious decision, every day, to notice the glimmers. There were endless difficult conversations, hours spent on the phone with doctors and piles of admin. There were big decisions to be made, and fraught conversations to be had. We missed my dad terribly during the Christmas festivities. But there was also, in stark contrast to that, the magical build-up to Christmas with kids who wholeheartedly believe in Father Christmas.

Is it possible to experience both/and? Both the heartache of an elderly parent entering his last chapter of life, and the delight of a child at the most wonderful time of the year? Perhaps that's life, as we grow older – we are all juggling so many different experiences, all at the same time. If we waited until it was all one or the other, we'd be immobilized. It is possible to move forward if you're looking for tiny moments of joy: thin slices that feel okay or even, sometimes, beautiful.

This is the power of crafting slices of joy and noticing glimmers – we had a Christmas filled with so many moments of joy. I still got to eat delicious food and play with my kids and revel in the magic of the season. If I hadn't been aware of slices of joy, I would have written the whole holiday off. Tiny glimmers saved me. They saved me because they were an anchor: I knew how important it was to hunt out the golden moments, even on the hard days.

My question to you is: what tiny thing could offer up a slice of joy for you today?

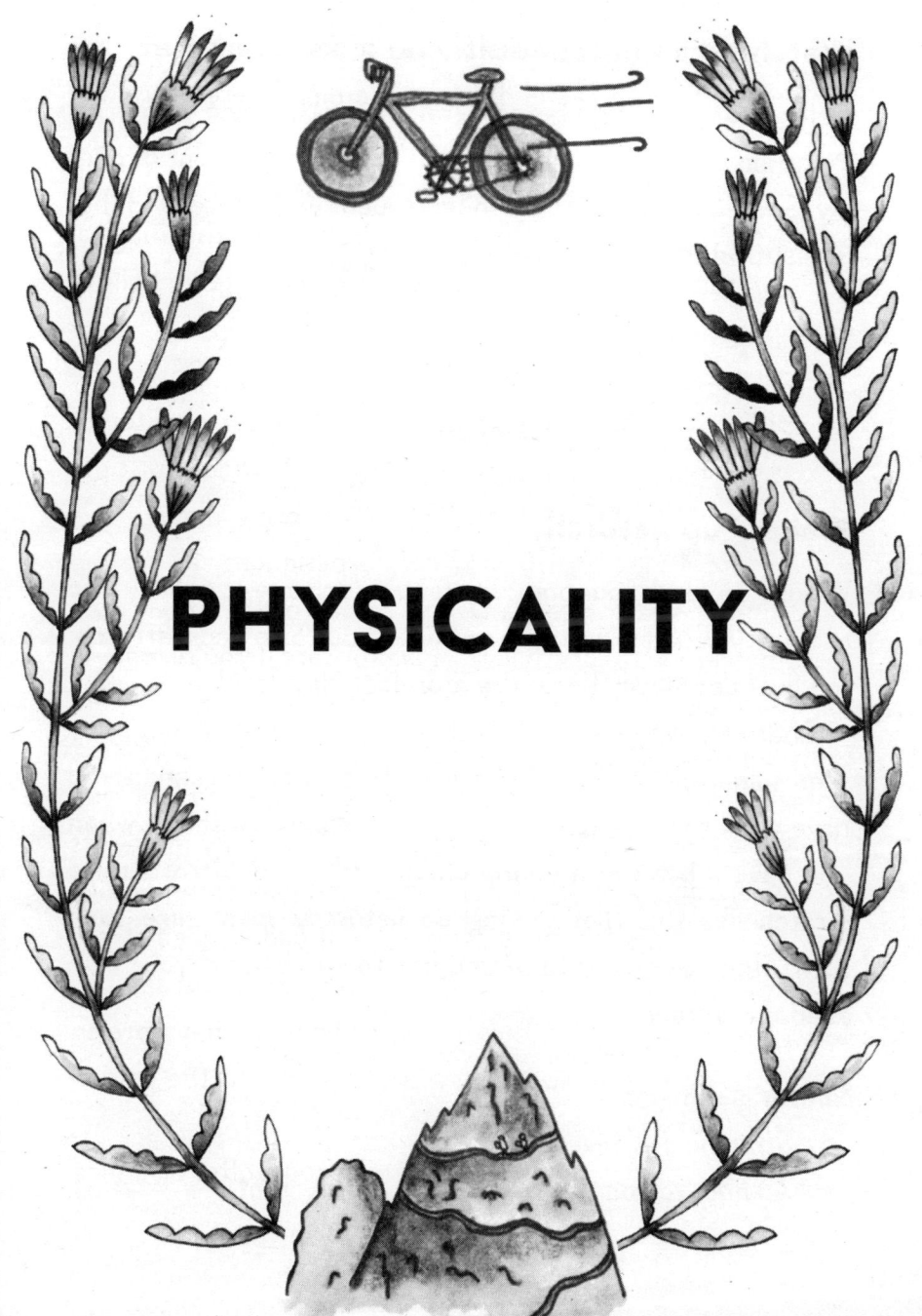

PHYSICALITY

Watching a kid (or adult!) do a dance of glee

A dance of glee could be a full-on dance, throwing your arms in the air, a little hip wiggle ... An unexpected moment of pure joy. Sometimes the whole dance happens in the face, and that is beautiful too.

Similar glimmers:
+ *Feeling playful.*
+ *Playing tag on a patch of grass.*

Waking up naturally

Waking up when your body wants to is such a gentle entry into the day. A chance to swim awake at your own pace, stretch, roll over and slowly begin the morning. How lovely.

There are whole stretches of life when waking up naturally seems an impossibility: If you have to do a school run, if you have work that starts early or you work unusual shifts, when you have a baby or a young child ... It's particularly after a stretch like this that waking up naturally seems like such a gift, but really any time you get to wake up of your own accord is a treat.

Similar glimmers:
+ *Stretching (streeeeeetching).*
+ *An hour to yourself to do whatever you want.*

The absence of pain

There have been many songs written about how you don't know what you've got 'til it's gone. I find that idea most striking when talking about pain, or illness of any kind. Here you are, merrily going about your life, unencumbered by headaches or vertigo or constant nausea, and unaware of how remarkable that is. But feeling normal is really the greatest gift ever. It's hard to appreciate the absence of something, it's true, but a few moments spent thinking about a time when you didn't feel well or strong can change the whole flavour of your day.

Similar glimmers:
+ *The relief of a headache lifting.*
+ *Taking off an uncomfortable outfit.*

Exercising until you feel your heart pumping

Isn't it remarkable that your heart is quietly pumping blood, without you having to do anything about it? Just pumping away, now, and now and now. It's only when you do some kind of intense exercise that you can actually feel your heart pumping, and that's a pretty remarkable thing too.

Similar glimmers:
+ *Hitting the magic zone on a run.*
+ *Breathing deeply after a week of a blocked nose.*

Dancing until your feet hurt

Adult life doesn't present that many occasions to dance the night away, unfortunately. But when the opportunity arises, and you can dance to music that you love until you're sweaty, out of breath and giddy with the thrill of being so present in your body, so vital and alive, it is a glorious thing.

A study at the University of Sydney showed that dancing can be more effective than other exercise at improving mental health.[9] That seems like a direct invitation to hunt down a kitchen dance party, a club or a dance class, doesn't it?

Similar glimmers:
+ *Running to music.*
+ *Punching a pillow (as hard as you can).*

Sleeping with the window open

Sleeping with the window open can offer such subtle joy ... the night sounds creeping in, the gentle breeze, the sense that stars and moonlight are not that far out of reach.

Similar glimmers:
+ *Walking in a forest, leaves crunching and the air smelling green.*
+ *The first asparagus/rhubarb/any other fruit or vegetable you anticipate of the season.*

Comfortable shoes

Perhaps it is only when you have worn dreadful shoes that you can truly appreciate the wonder of comfortable shoes. In my first year of college in the USA, I wore red suede clogs in a city that snowed for months. Another year I wore boots I absolutely loved, but they were a size too small. Ouch.

Now that I am a wise old woman, I deeply value the sense of security and safety a comfortable pair of shoes can offer. They can't be too ugly, of course (I still have standards!) but a comfortable pair of shoes can turn a long day into a manageable one.

Similar glimmers:
+ *The perfect boots for the weather: your feet dry as you walk through puddles.*
+ *The first day it's warm enough to walk around without shoes or socks on.*

Sex

Consensual, loving and in your own time.

Similar glimmers:
+ *Kissing. It's such a shortcut to feeling like a teenager again, lips bruised and head filled with cotton wool.*
+ *A hug where you fit together.*

Breathing deeply

Take a deep breath. And exhale. Deep belly breaths are pretty much guaranteed to make you feel better.

When is the last time you remembered to breathe deeply? It can be weirdly easy to go through a whole day shallow breathing, especially if you're working hunched over a desk. On days that are particularly hard, one conscious breath in, and then out, can be your slice of joy.

Similar glimmers:
+ *Feeling abundantly well and full of beans.*
+ *Laughing so hard you can't catch your breath between rounds of laughter.*

Stroking a purring cat

The way the purring seems to resonate throughout their whole furry body and into your hand and thereby into you. The deep and profound comfort. The love.

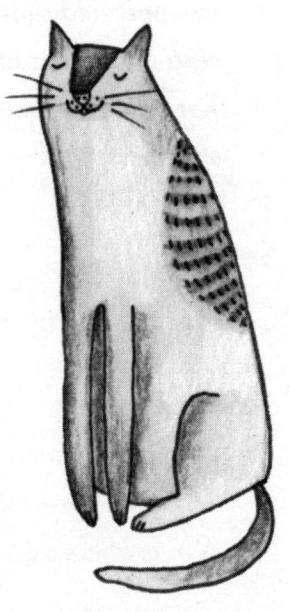

Similar glimmers:
+ *Watching a dog chase its tail.*
+ *Throwing a stick (or a ball) for a dog: the glee!*

Falling asleep easily

Sleep is the new sex, apparently.[10] I can believe it. Modern life – with all its devices and demands and constant, unending grasping at what little shreds of attention you have left – has made sleep something rather elusive and somewhat difficult to hold onto.

Falling asleep easily has become a rare skill. So when it happens, when sleep steals over you while you're reading and makes you drop your book, or your head hits the pillow and sleep knocks you out, oh! What deliciousness that is.

Similar glimmers:
+ *An unhurried shower. So often you have to hurriedly jump in and out of the shower, but on the rare occasion that you can luxuriate in the falling water, well! Isn't that just wonderful?*
+ *Resting under a tree: nowhere to go, nothing to do.*

Getting clean after sweaty exercise

Your body temperature rises and you start sweating. And then you get to cool down: whether it's a swim or a shower, it is tingly and delightful to get clean after physical exertion. It also helps your heart rate reduce, and ensures you'll be more palatable to other people because you won't be a sweaty mess. But the true joy of getting clean after a workout is the way it feels.

Similar glimmers:
+ *The first swim in the ocean/swimming pool/natural body of water of the season.*
+ *Laughing until you cry or your sides ache.*

Heat on a sore muscle

Many people are nursing a sore muscle of some description – tight shoulders from working too hard, sore feet from standing all day ... Isn't it such a relief to tend to the ache? Whether it's a microwave hot sack, a heated pad or hot water from the shower pummelling away the tension, that sense of ease when you apply heat and the pain dissolves a little is visceral.

Similar glimmers:
+ *Tingly legs after a long walk.*
+ *Doing some kind of physical labour (lifting, carrying, gardening ...) until your muscles ache pleasantly.*

Having your hair washed in a salon

If you don't mind strangers touching you, a scalp massage and/or hair wash before a haircut is one of the few times that you can just lie back, relax and let someone else care for you. For a few glorious minutes. No guilt, no To Do List, just ... exhale.

Similar glimmers:
+ *Freshly dyed hair.*
+ *Fingernails at the perfect length for you.*

Feeling hunger pangs – and then eating

There is a real joy to be found in not eating until you're hungry: properly hungry. Waiting to feel hunger pangs, and then eating. "Hunger is the best sauce," my mom always used to say, suggesting (I think) that when you're hungry, food tastes better. Want to give it a try today?

Similar glimmers:
+ *Making time to savour your food. Whether it's eating a quick lunch in front of your computer or wolfing down dinner because it's late and you're tired, so many meals seem to rush past without proper attention. Taking time to sit and eat, with no other distractions, is a real joy.*
+ *Cracking open a cold drink (can or bottle).*

A quiet street when everyone is still asleep

Super-early morning feels almost mystical: when anyone sensible is still tucked up in bed but for whatever reason you find yourself in a car or bus or on foot, moving past all the sleeping houses.

Similar glimmers:
+ *Browsing the stacks at a library.*
+ *Going to a show at a planetarium (and being reminded how tiny you really are, in the greater cosmos).*

Church bells, particularly at dusk

Their song sings out across the village or town or city, signalling that it is Time. It doesn't really matter what it's Time for, simply that this, now, deserves marking. Just for a moment.

In the pause, there is listening: to the bells, yes, but also to the moment, and your body in it.

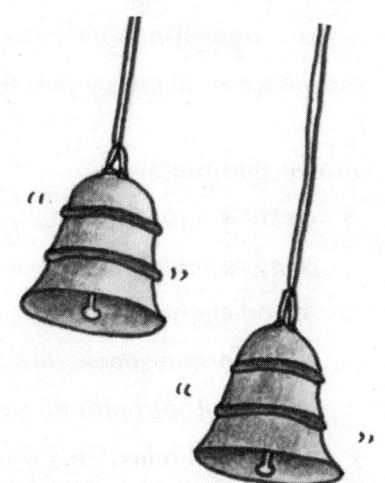

Similar glimmers:
+ *Silence so loud it sings.*
+ *Finding the exact right alarm tone to wake you up.*

Being out of your comfort zone in a thrilling way

Being slightly out of your comfort zone, somewhere that is starkly beautiful or difficult to reach in normal life, somewhere that perhaps doesn't offer all the creature comforts you're used to, but lets you see life from a different perspective.

Similar glimmers:
+ *Snorkelling – all that colour! All that life!*
+ *Kayaking on a river and feeling the oar slice through the water.*

Watching the world go by from a train

There is life to be lived and things to do, but for now all you need to do is gaze out of the window at the rolling scenery. Homes, skyscrapers, fields, forests, roads ... it doesn't really matter, because there's nothing you have to do but sit back and watch it all pass you by.

Similar glimmers:
+ *Letting a foreign language wash over you: no idea what they're saying but it sure sounds beautiful, doesn't it?*
+ *Candlelight. It's almost magical the way candles can transform a space ... The gently flickering flames, the dim lighting that hides all the clutter, the invitation to slow down and relax.*

"I love this song!"

It's almost a physical jolt. You're walking through a store when your favourite song suddenly starts playing, and something in you leaps. Or you have your phone playing a thousand songs on shuffle and one pops up that is absolutely perfect for this moment, right now. Or you're with friends, chatting, when the background music suddenly becomes foreground because you love the song that's playing. What a surprise. What a delight!

Music is a shortcut to nostalgia and memory, but it's also a shortcut to feeling great, even if it's only for three minutes while the song is playing.

Similar glimmers:
+ *A chair stretch: arms reaching for the ceiling, spine popping back into place.*
+ *Climbing a tree (that's easy to climb). You swing up, experimentally, to the first branch. Then, like a ladder climbing up to the heavens, you keep climbing. What joy! What freedom! What a thrill to be perched above the world.*

A fast walk on a cool morning

You've seen those people. You've been those people. Striding along as if your legs could carry you all day long. It's a feeling of bottled power and vitality, made all the more poignant because so many people struggle to stride, for any number of reasons. When the stride hits you, hold onto it with both hands and thank it for coming your way.

Similar glimmers:

+ *Yoga or Pilates or any other exercise that stretches you in ways you didn't know you could.*
+ *Running for the bus and catching it, when you thought you were too late.*

A full fridge

Opening the door to a full fridge remains one of the great joys of being an adult, in my opinion. Not over-full, mind you, I don't want to have to start worrying about food going bad. But a nicely stocked fridge, offering up various possibilities for meals without me having to think too hard or get too creative in the leftovers department feels like a pretty big gift.

Similar glimmers:

+ *Lying on a heated massage table.*
+ *The scent of freshly-baked anything.*

Riding a bicycle downhill

As adults, there aren't that many opportunities for that giddy sense of safety-fear (you know, when you're technically safe, but you still feel a tinge of fear from the speed at which you're moving). It can be a helpful reminder that you are, actually, very alive and, in fact, very much a body with a mind, rather than the other way around. Down you fly! Wind in your hair!

Similar glimmers:
+ *Going down a slide.*
+ *The joy/terror combo of a fairground ride.*

Creature comforts

I am not a natural camper. I like a bed and a private shower. But when I have willingly camped, one of my favourite things is coming home to an electric kettle and a beautifully made bed, and a bathroom that I don't have to share with anyone. Even just imagining a camping trip can make me grateful for my creature comforts, which feels like a double win.

Similar glimmers:
+ *Stepping out of a cold, icy wind into shelter. And all of a sudden it stops. There is stillness, warmth and relief.*
+ *Watching really hard rain pelt a window when you're cosy and dry inside. Extra points if there's also thunder.*

Taking a dog off leash in a wide open space

If you ever need a visible definition of the word "vitality", it's a dog who is desperate to run being let off their leash. There they go – a streak of movement across the wide open space. It's a giddy experience to watch that much bottled-up energy being unleashed all at once.

Similar glimmers:
+ *Coming home to a dog so happy to see you their whole torso wags.*
+ *Watching birds at a full bird feeder.*

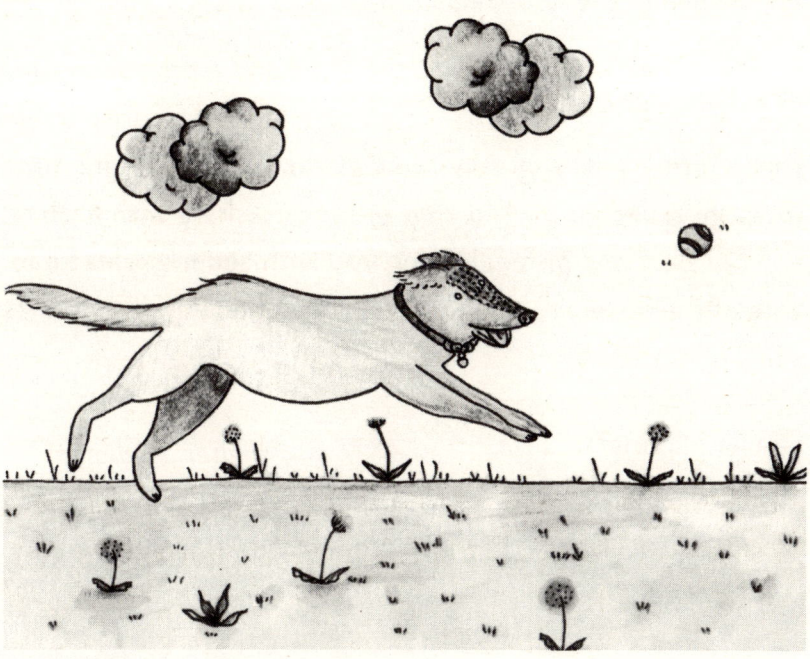

Whizzing along at speed

If you spend any time around kids, you'll notice that they hardly ever walk. Instead, they run or skip or hop or gambol. Somehow, adults almost inevitably and always walk. And it's at a measured pace! How dull.

So when opportunities present themselves to fly – like when you're riding a bicycle on a long, straight road, and you can really whip yourself up to a heady speed – they are such a balm to the child who's trapped inside wanting to frolic more.

Similar glimmers:
+ *Swinging on a swing – higher! Higher!*
+ *Skipping. Even one skip in the middle of a normal walk.*

Washing your hair

That slightly gritty, greasy feeling when you know it's time to wash your hair ... And that glorious sudsing and washing away of dust and grime, leaving you with squeaky clean hair. One of the fastest routes to feeling better, even if it only lasts a few minutes.

Similar glimmers:
+ *A fresh towel after a bath or shower.*
+ *Hugging someone you love who you haven't seen for a long time.*

Unconditional love from your pet

In a world filled with uncertainty, a pet can offer the most stable, unconditional love. Always there, ready for a cuddle, delighted to see you and happy to curl up in your lap. They don't argue or demand more than their due; they merely offer a daily dose of love and joy.

Similar glimmers:
+ *Feeding a pet their favourite snack.*
+ *The way playing with a pet brings you directly into the present moment: totally focused on the now.*

A full body massage

You go in a stressed-out ball of knotted muscles, and emerge as pliable as a piece of cooked spaghetti. Human touch can be such a gift. When is the last time you had a massage, or your equivalent delight? Any chance you could find a gap for one this week?

Similar glimmers:
+ *A bear hug. One of those where you are completely enveloped by the other person and so happy to just live in that moment for a few breaths.*
+ *A foot rub, when all the tension just melts away.*

An already-unpacked dishwasher

It's another thing to complete before you can finally sit down and relax ... You open the dishwasher, ready to start unpacking it and find ... Oh, wonder of wonders! It's been unpacked already!

It seems like such a small thing, but it's like a helping hand has reached out and patted you, gently, on the back.

Similar glimmers:
+ *Vacuuming with a powerful vacuum cleaner.*
+ *A hot shower on a cold morning: instant comfort.*

Brushing your hair at the end of the day

Or whatever your end of day rhythm entails. Something that is soothing, repetitive and signals to your body that now it's time to rest.

Similar glimmers:
+ *Stepping outside into the cool, still evening.*
+ *Walking up a hill and looking back at how far you've come.*

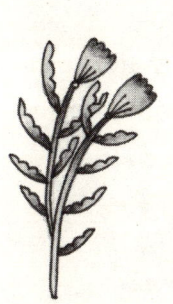

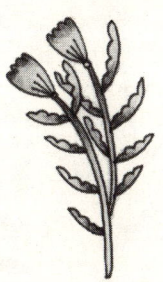

THE TINIEST THING CAN BE A GLIMMER

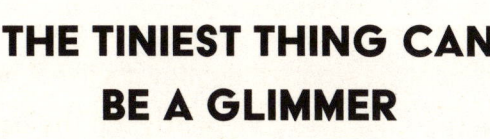

At the end of the day, cast your mind back and sift through what happened. Was there anything a little bit shiny that sticks out, anything that glimmers?

+ Maybe connecting with other people?
+ Something sensory that felt really nice?
+ Did you eat or drink anything tasty?
+ Perhaps something at work: did you manage to complete a project that felt satisfying, or did a meeting go well?
+ If all else fails, how was the weather today? Any glimmers there?

Remember that you're looking for tiny slivers of light here. Anything that felt nice. Nice! Not awesome or amazing or fabulous or spectacular or even lovely. Simply nice.

What's one glimmer of joy from today?

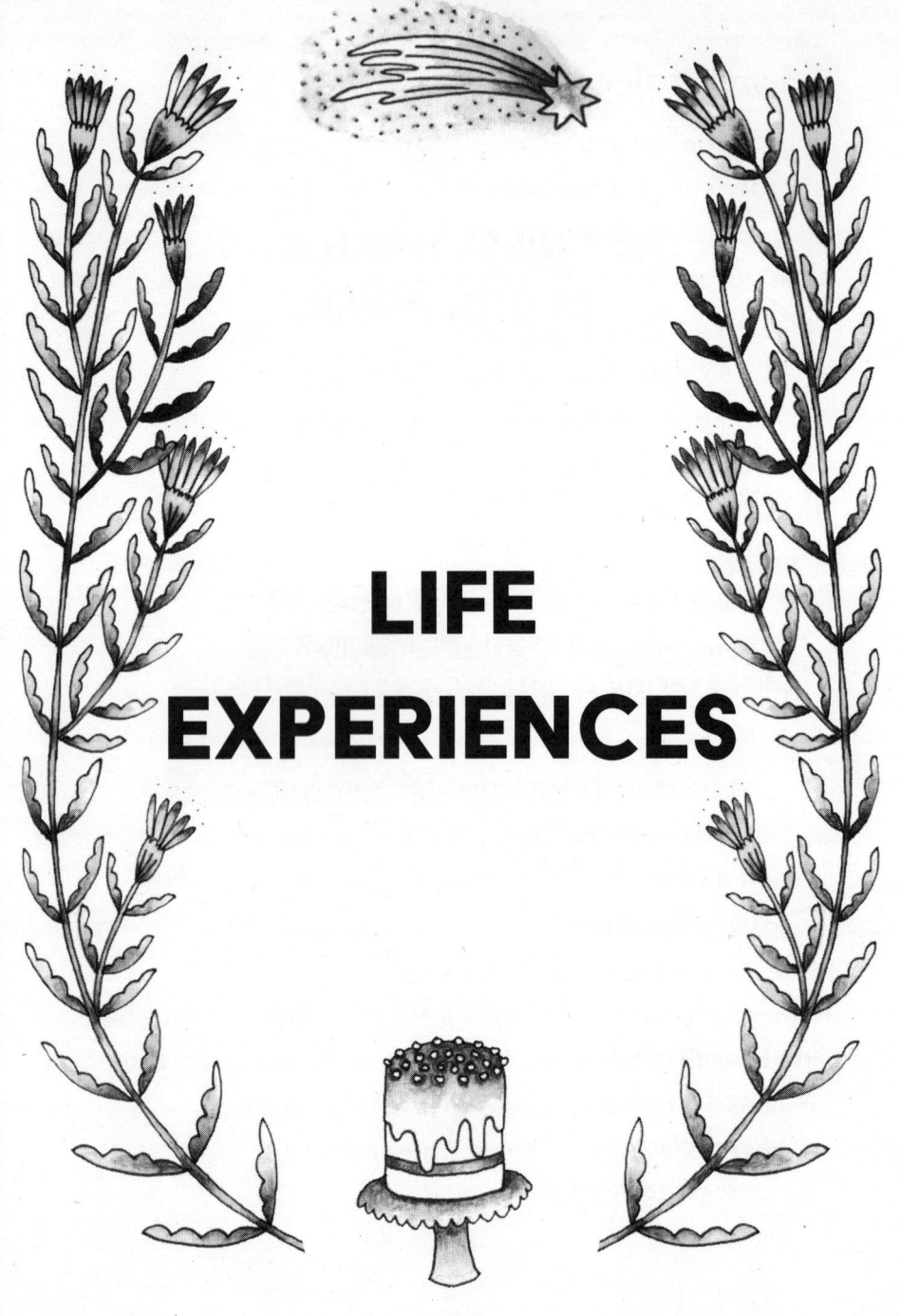

LIFE
EXPERIENCES

A familiar view, seen anew

You know when you've been away from home for a few days, and then you return to your neighbourhood, and it's as if you're seeing it all for the first time? Maybe your view is prettier than you remembered, or your street is more charming, the trees are in leaf, or everything is simply imbued with such familiarity that you know you're home, again.

Similar glimmers:
+ *Waking up at your usual time, the day after a super-early wake-up call.*
+ *Returning to a beloved restaurant after an absence.*

Rediscovering a song from your youth

From the moment the opening chords play, you're transported back: to your teens, or your twenties, or whenever you listened to this song so many times the lyrics burnt themselves into your brain. It's not that you want to return there, exactly, but it's such a treat to revisit that younger self, and remember how you used to feel.

Similar glimmers:
+ *Rediscovering childhood toys.*
+ *Rewatching a TV show or film you loved when you were younger (and it's still great!).*

Creating (anything)

Baking something, making a card, writing some words, drawing a picture, sewing a little something, building Lego, writing code, singing a tune you just made up, or any of the other myriad ways humans can be creative. Creating something (anything) is a glorious feeling.

Who cares if it's any good? Nobody has to see it. The whole point is in the magic of using your hands and your imagination to make something that wasn't there before.

Similar glimmers:
+ *Co-creating (something fun or meaningful) with other people.*
+ *Art projects with no rules.*

Getting a free gift with a purchase

It doesn't really matter what it is. For me, it's the thrill of getting something new and surprising (and totally free!). Bonus points if it's something cool, but even if you immediately regift or donate it, it's nice to be given a little glimmer on an otherwise ordinary day.

Similar glimmers:
+ *Receiving an unanticipated gift ("For me?! Thank you!").*
+ *An item you need (or want) on sale or in a thrift store.*

Being in the zone

Being in the zone is the best feeling. The sense that you could fly through whatever it is you're doing, and not have to touch the ground. It happens when you give yourself space and time, stay focused but not too focused, have good snacks available so you don't have to stop, and know how to do whatever it is you're doing. It's glorious! Fleeting, intangible, but glorious.

Similar glimmers:
+ *A great idea.*
+ *Reading a poem aloud that hits the spot.*

Beautiful design

So much of life is functional, and if not ugly, then certainly not beautiful. That's why really good design – design that takes the form and function and aesthetics of the whole into account and creates something both clever and subtle – is such a treat. You'll know it's good design when it gives you a feeling of peace and satisfaction at the same time. Like a beautifully made bowl or an amazing architectural building. Mastery made tangible.

Similar glimmers:
+ *Finishing an excellent book.*
+ *Street art that surprises and delights you.*

Snapshot moments

In the olden days, special moments would have been captured on camera and printed out for the photo album or the fridge. These days, they're more likely to end up on Instagram or sent to your close friends or family. These are the snapshot moments: the ones when everything aligns, for a moment or two, and you want to commemorate it because it is so unusual and lovely. It might simply be two friends together, or a beautiful view that made you feel hopeful ... something worth remembering in the moment.

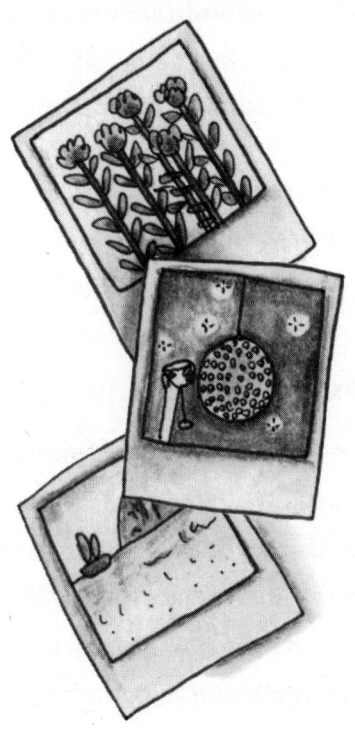

Similar glimmers:
+ *Eating an ice cream while walking somewhere pretty.*
+ *Building an epic sandcastle.*

Finding exactly what you're looking for

What are the odds? You know exactly what you'd love – the cut, the colour, the size – but how likely are you to actually find it? And then you do! And it's as if all the gods in shopping heaven conspired simply to offer you this garment, as a reward for doing your best every day.

Similar glimmers:
+ *Perfectly sharpened pencils.*
+ *When you break something you love and find a replacement that's as good – or even better.*

Being awake (on purpose) in a sleeping house

There's nothing worse than desperately wanting to be asleep and instead roaming around your home like a sleepless ghost. But the flip side of that is being purposefully awake – either late at night or early in the morning – while everyone else sleeps. There's such stillness, such peace, such a sense of "anything could happen" (in the nicest possible way).

Similar glimmers:
+ *Eating a food from childhood that tastes exactly how you remember it.*
+ *Watching whatever you want on TV, without having to negotiate with anyone.*

An uneventful health check-up

It might not be the most exciting slice of joy, but going for a health check-up and finding nothing wrong is something to celebrate. Imagine all the various ways your body could fail you. All the many tiny and big things that could go wrong? And you, lucky, miraculous you, are just fine.

What a relief. What a blessing.

Similar glimmers:
+ *An afternoon stroll around the block.*
+ *Golden sun through the car or bus window.*

Dinner and a movie

There are times in life for grand adventures, but there are also times for small, beautiful ordinary adventures. Like dinner and a movie.

Remember lockdown? When the whole world shut down in the grips of a pandemic? When there was true longing to meet a friend for dinner, in an actual restaurant? Or the thought of sitting in a cinema with strangers, all breathing the same air was inconceivable? And now! Look at us now.

Similar glimmers:
+ *A coffee shop with good, free WiFi.*
+ *Favourite take-out, favourite couch.*

Clearing out

You've been meaning to do it for ages, and you finally tackle that cupboard. What a joy to get rid of things you no longer need or want! There's a sense of freedom in having extra space, and in seeing the things you care about become uncluttered.

The second joy lies in giving items to someone else – perhaps a charity store or a friend. Watching an unwanted item get a chance at a second life is a total slice of joy.

Similar glimmers:
+ *Benefitting from someone else clearing out. A toy for your child or a book you've been wanting to read.*
+ *Wiping down a countertop that has crumbs and sticky spilt stuff on it until it gleams.*

Spending a gift voucher

There are some people who feel that a gift voucher isn't a thoughtful gift, but I am not one of them. I absolutely love a gift voucher: it's like being given pretend money that can be spent on whatever you choose! What fun.

Similar glimmers:
+ *Exploring a small local store.*
+ *Leaving a store wearing something you just bought because you love it so much.*

A water pistol fight

When is the last time you had a water pistol fight? Any chance you could initiate one sometime this week?

There's no need for a whole cavalry: it can simply be a two-person water pistol fight, somewhere outdoors, close to home for when you get wet and want to change into dry clothes. But oh! The fun. The wild wonderfulness of shooting water at someone, and trying to dodge the water that comes shooting back at you.

Similar glimmers:
+ *Riding a carousel (and getting to choose your animal!).*
+ *An unexpected flower delivery.*

A tea party

Preferably with fancy tea cups and teeny tiny cakes and tarts, but let's be honest, any tea party will do. It's the ritual of it: the fuss and unnecessary prettiness that makes it so special. But it's also about marking time, right? Not just brushing today under the carpet as Another Day, but giving it a little gold dust to make it feel special.

Similar glimmers:
+ *An impromptu dance party in your kitchen.*
+ *Someone making you a birthday cake.*

Celebrating a half-birthday

There is not often cause for celebration as adults. Have you noticed? Even birthdays aren't as big a deal as they used to be, and there hasn't been much of a replacement celebration, in my opinion, except for the Big Things such as weddings, graduations and babies.

In light of this, I'd like to suggest that you celebrate your half-birthdays. It can be with something minor: half a cake perhaps, or your favourite snack, or choosing exactly what you want for dinner. One little way to mark your halfway journey round the sun.

Similar glimmers:

+ *Framing a picture you love (a photo, a sketch, a scribble ...).*
+ *Going out for dessert or ice cream.*

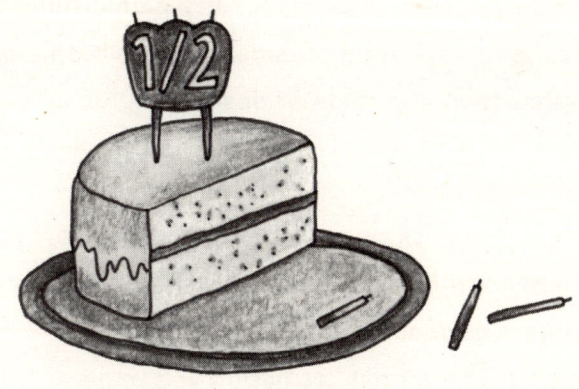

Getting dressed up

Making an effort with your appearance is special; it's a reminder that you're as young as you'll ever be, and you might as well enjoy it. Even if you feel a little awkward in fancy clothes, odds are you'll be glad you did it (think how comfortable your normal clothes will feel tomorrow!).

Similar glimmers:
+ *Popping the cork on a bottle of bubbly (alcoholic or non-alcoholic, it doesn't make a difference).*
+ *Feeling celebratory. The giddy sense of glee in the room, the fizz in the atmosphere.*

A picnic

Ideally a waterside picnic in dappled sunshine, with a quilted picnic blanket and a wicker basket filled with organic, homemade delicacies ... But really, any picnic will do. It's so liberating to take your food outside, and eat it on a bench or blanket, rather than at a table or desk.

Similar glimmers:
+ *Day trips. You pack up your things and head off for a little mini adventure. Home before the day is over but oh! A change is as good as a holiday.*
+ *Going to a local tourist attraction you've never been to.*

Appreciating a sunset

Isn't it remarkable that the sun sets every day? It's hard to pay it any heed, most of the time, because it's hidden behind clouds or buildings, but think of a time when you were on holiday somewhere and really appreciated the sunset. Watched it go down, waited until the last embers of fiery sun had slipped below the horizon ... Remember that? Could you find a moment sometime this week to pause and appreciate the sunset?

Similar glimmers:
+ *Toasting marshmallows over a fire (indoor or outdoor).*
+ *Staring into an open fire, watching the flames dance.*

Winning a prize

It's not even about the prize, is it? It could be a tombola or a local competition with a hamper of some kind filled with fairly ordinary things. That's not what matters. What matters is being the lucky one, chosen from so many, to be a winner! That little glow can light up a whole day.

Similar glimmers:
+ *The giddy overwhelm of a carnival.*
+ *Picking fresh flowers or fruit.*

A solo cinema date

It can feel absolutely thrilling to go to the cinema on your own, especially in the middle of the day. The movie you want to watch isn't necessarily the same as your partner or friend, so why insist on going together? It's far better to see the movie you want to, undisturbed. Bonus points are that you don't have to share your popcorn!

Similar glimmers:
+ *Listening to your favourite music, turned up loud.*
+ *Going to the theatre or a gig on your own.*

Reading a book outside

It's the very picture of leisure, isn't it? Lying down reading in your garden. It can just as easily be a magazine or a tablet or your phone, and it doesn't have to be a garden if you prefer a park, the beach or a city bench. It's the act of gifting yourself some time to read whatever it is you love reading (novel, poem, news, gossip mag) and getting some fresh air at the same time.

Similar glimmers:
+ *People-watching in a public space: little stories unfolding on all sides.*
+ *Going for a walk outside to clear your head.*

Mastery

There is mastery on display everywhere – it's in the beautifully timed traffic lights that keep traffic flowing smoothly, the teacher guiding schoolkids along a busy street, the treats in the bakery window, the banker deftly counting out notes ...

It is rarely noticed purely because we are used to things running so smoothly. Like a giant silent orchestra being conducted invisibly behind the scenes.

Similar glimmers:

✦ *Synchronicity: When things line up just exactly as they should, and fall into place in a way that feels like there must be a puppet master behind the scenes. You run into an acquaintance who mentions a job opening that's exactly what you're looking for, and applications close in a week. Uncanny!*

✦ *Shared awe: That surge of energy that lifts you and everyone else around you up. Usually experienced while watching a performance of some kind or in the presence of extraordinary natural beauty.*

The glee of trying something new

There is delight in trying something new that you enjoy. It's a reminder that you are alive, and growing new neural pathways every day. Even if so much of life is predictable, there are still many new adventures to be had! Micro adventures, perhaps, but adventures nonetheless. It could be trying your hand at a painting class, learning a new language, or working out how to fix something. Well done, you!

Similar glimmers:
+ *Skimming stones.*
+ *Discovering a new café or store in your neighbourhood.*

Exciting shoes

The definition of "exciting" is entirely up to you – maybe the shoes are your favourite brand or maybe they're in a jazzy colour. Maybe they're covered in rainbow sequins that catch the light with every step you take. No judgement here!

Walking around in exciting shoes is particularly fun because in many other ways you're just going about your daily business … It's like carrying a little bit of magic on your feet.

Similar glimmers:
+ *Fancy fingernails (like tiny works of art).*
+ *Wearing beautiful underwear.*

A perfectly dark bedroom at night

Each person is so specific, and unique. There has literally never been another you! That blows my mind. There are certain things you like, and don't like, and some things that bring you great pleasure and others that drive you nuts: it's not always that easy to predict what those are going to be. For me, the perfect darkness in my bedroom at night is a source of great comfort. It is so sweet. What is that special thing for you?

Similar glimmers:
+ *A shower that ticks all the boxes: right temperature, right pressure, right duration.*
+ *Finishing a task exactly the way you want to.*

Nostalgia

Nostalgia, by its very nature, is bittersweet. It's remembering something that fills your heart with both sweetness and an ache. But there's a glimmer of joy in nostalgia, and it can be such fun to take a wander down memory lane, even if it's only for a few minutes.

Similar glimmers:
+ *Looking through old photos of happy times.*
+ *Stumbling across a forgotten video clip from the past.*

Really dressing up for a fancy dress party

Have you noticed that as you get older, it's more acceptable to not really be into things? You can get away with half-baked enthusiasm and not diving in whole-heartedly. I suppose it's seen as growing up? I disagree with this profoundly. We should all be diving whole-heartedly into the things we care about!

So, if you're going to a dress-up party: Dress. Up. If you really love the way someone does something: Tell. Them. And if you want to emphasize how you feel about a certain issue: Capitalize. Each. Word.

Similar glimmers:
+ *Putting up decorations to celebrate pretty much any occasion.*
+ *Taking the time to present a meal beautifully: your best plates, a little sprinkling of herbs, candlelight and the nice cutlery.*

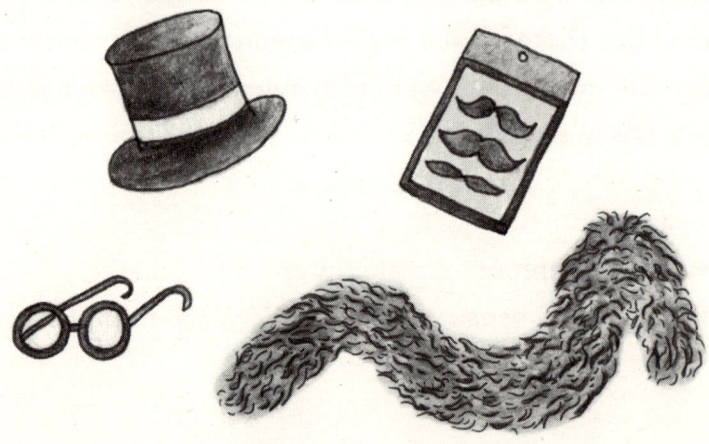

A tidy home

Every so often, the heavens shower you with blessings and your home looks the way you want it to. The clutter has been tidied away, the dishes are washed and stacked, all is peaceful and calm and tidy. Depending on your life situation, this may be a daily reality or a once-a-year occurrence, but it's worth pausing and noticing how beautiful it is when you chance upon it.

Similar glimmers:
+ *Being at home alone (when the house is usually full of people).*
+ *The calm after guests leave.*

Having someone cook you dinner

We all have to eat dinner every day, so it shouldn't be such a surprise that someone has to cook it. But when it's cooked for you – preferably with love, enthusiasm and organic ingredients, but let's not be fussy! – it feels like a real treat. Whether it's first date territory, or years down the line, having someone cook you dinner is so special.

Similar glimmers:
+ *Having someone read poetry or funny rhymes out loud.*
+ *Someone else making the bed.*

Surprise good news

I begin every morning with a version of Piglet's timeless question: "I wonder what's going to happen exciting today?"

Most days there's nothing particularly surprising, but on those occasions that there really is surprise good news, I double down on it. I relish its delicious unexpectedness and tell anyone who might care. It can be so easy to downplay the good, for fear of ... what, exactly? Making other people feel bad? But in truth, most of the time I've found that others are delighted to share in your good fortune. There isn't always that much of it to go around.

Similar glimmers:

+ *Opening a beautifully wrapped present. The whole process: untying the bow, carefully or not-carefully unsticking the tape, carefully or not-carefully taking the paper off and then! Voila! The big reveal!*
+ *Hearing good news from someone you love.*

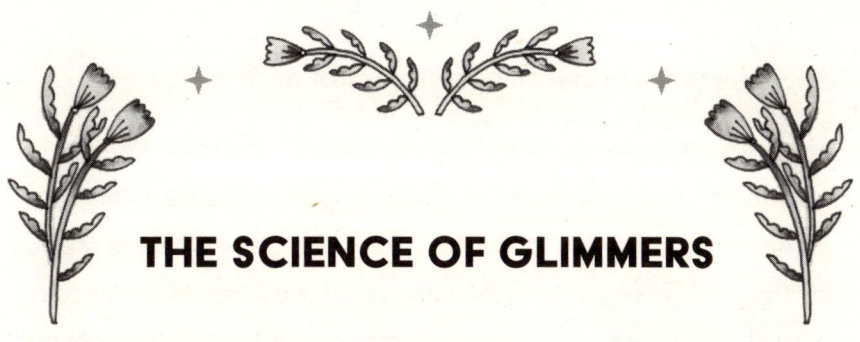

THE SCIENCE OF GLIMMERS

Joy isn't just an airy-fairy feeling; it has tangible, scientific effects on our mind and body, with specific effects on our wellbeing. The American Psychological Association (APA) describes joy like this:

JOY: *noun.*

A feeling of extreme gladness, delight, or exaltation of the spirit arising from a sense of wellbeing or satisfaction. The feeling of joy may take two forms: passive and active.[11]

Sounds pretty good, right? But extreme gladness, delight or exaltation of the spirit seem quite exhausting ... Wellbeing and satisfaction, though? Yes, please.

The APA goes on to describe passive joy as the tranquil, content type of joy. Active joy spices things up by involving other people. Active joy might be more intense, but both forms are positively associated with an increase in energy, confidence and self-esteem. That means that a focus on joy brings us more energy, and empowers us to feel more confident as we move through the world. If you weren't already convinced that this is a worthy practice, that should do it!

✦ Advice from the happiest person on the planet

Matthieu Ricard is the French writer, photographer and Buddhist monk known as "the happiest person on the planet".[12] Ricard got that title after a 12-year medical study at the University of Wisconsin, in which they did rigorous neurological tests on their subjects, so it's probably a pretty sound assessment, but still. Honestly, what a moniker. What if you're having a really bad day? How do you square that with being the happiest person on the planet?

What's interesting is that Ricard thinks that "happiness" is too vague a term: he prefers "wellbeing". Ricard adds that, "the best definition, according to the Buddhist view, is that wellbeing is not just a mere pleasurable sensation. It is a deep sense of serenity and fulfilment."

So, rather than wanting happiness, let's take the advice and aim, instead, for wellbeing.

Wellbeing becomes the soil from which slices of joy can grow. It is intrinsically linked to mindfulness: an awareness of your life as it happens, as opposed to being lost in movies of the past or projections of the future. The whole idea is to notice your life, right here, right now. To appreciate this bite of crunchy apple, or this comfortable cushion in exactly the right place on your back, or this soft shirt caressing your skin. And once the moment is gone, that's it. No grasping, no trying to hang onto things, simply appreciating this, right now.

✦ Wellbeing and the nervous system

I have recently become fascinated by the nervous system, and how it relates to joy and everyday life. I've found that a greater awareness of my nervous system has made life in general much easier to deal with. That feeling of being frazzled (you know what I mean) is really your parasympathetic nervous system needing some care.

Research has shown that joy activates the parasympathetic nervous system (linked to feelings of peace and calm), while happiness activates the sympathetic nervous system (linked to excitement, energy and activity).[13]

Joy is felt in our neurotransmitters, the tiny chemical cells that transmit messages between neurons (our nerves) and other cells in the body.[14] The physical sense of joy that we experience is the result of two types of neurotransmitters: dopamine (the feel-good hormone) and serotonin (the mood stabilizer hormone). These are known as the "happy hormones", along with oxytocin (the love hormone) and endorphins (the exercise hormone). Dopamine and serotonin, in particular, are closely associated with happiness. They are often in short supply in those dealing with clinical depression.

Emma Suttie, an acupuncture physician writing in *The Epoch Times*, takes it one step further, saying that, "joy is a healthy mental state that promotes our internal organs' effective functioning and a balanced emotional state. Joy makes the mind peaceful and relaxed, benefits the immune system, and causes the body to relax and slow down."[15]

A healthy mental state that causes the body to relax and slow down ... We can all benefit from that.

✦ Sources of joy

There are two kinds of joy: eudaimonic and hedonic.[16] Both have their roots in ancient Greece, and they look at the source of joy:

1. Eudaimonic wellbeing most often springs from things that bring you meaning and authenticity. So, eudaimonic pursues meaning as a route to joy. You'll notice this kind of joy when you're helping a friend, or learning something new. It's closely aligned with satisfaction.

2. Hedonic wellbeing offers you immediate hits of pleasure (maximizing pleasure and minimizing displeasure). So, hedonic pursues pleasure as a route to joy. A dance party or a fabulous slice of cake can offer you hedonic wellbeing.

One is not better than the other, and we need a blend of both for a balanced life. You'll notice that these two kinds of joy don't map exactly on to the two forms of joy – active and passive – because pursuing meaning can be tranquil or intense, solo or with others, as can pleasure.

Joy, then, is a unique blend: connecting with the things that truly, deeply mean something to you: physically, mentally, emotionally (eudaimonic wellbeing). And, on the flip side, things that bring you immediate pleasure, for a minute or two (hedonic wellbeing).

Most of all, though, joy is recognizing that the small, simple things carry great power. Iris Murdoch once said: "People from a planet without flowers would think we must be mad with joy the whole time to have such things about us."[17]

Yes! Why aren't we?

Murdoch also said, "One of the secrets of a happy life is continuous small treats," and if that's not an invitation to go and get yourself a small treat right now, I don't know what is.

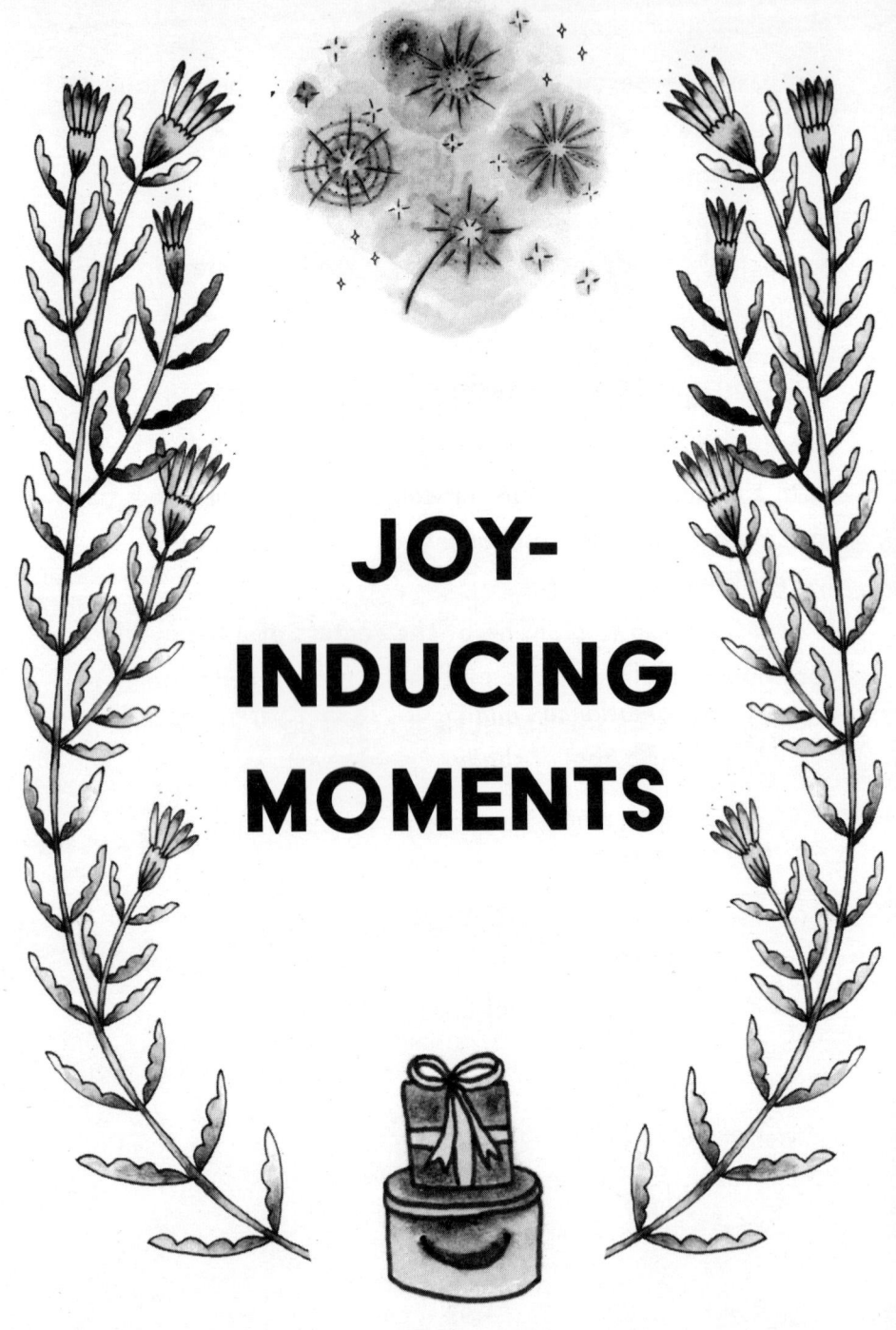

JOY-INDUCING MOMENTS

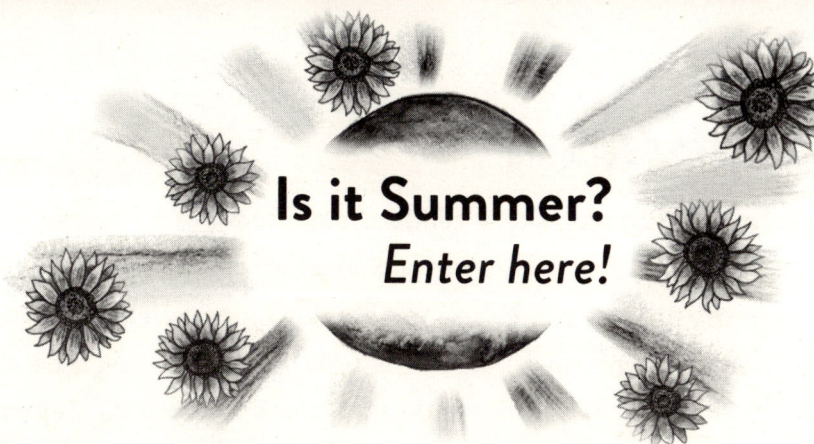

Is it Summer?
Enter here!

Stepping into the shade on a sunny day

Your eyes take a moment to adjust as you step from the sun into the shade. Your skin almost instantly cools, and your mind exhales as everything recalibrates to a slightly less bright version of itself.

Similar glimmers:

+ *An air-conditioned building or vehicle on a hot day.*
+ *An umbrella pool of shade.*

An outdoor movie

An outdoor movie feels both retro – back to the days of drive-in cinemas – and extremely chic. Look at you, lounging outdoors watching a movie! Living your best life.

Similar glimmers:

+ *A silly movie that makes you laugh out loud.*
+ *A music festival, as the night draws in.*

A jar of delights

There's nothing like a random day (today?) to start a new tradition. How about getting a clean jar, filling it with 52 empty slips of paper, and writing down one lovely thing each week, for the next year? This time next year, you'll be able to look back at all the wonderful little things that happened to you ... It's a homegrown jar of gratitude.

Similar glimmers:
+ *A new cookbook.*
+ *Being reminded of photos and memories from this day last year (as if by phone magic!).*

Swimming in the sea before breakfast

The glee comes from the sheer joy of doing something unexpected and fun before the day begins. You might prefer a morning run, a mountain walk or rowing a boat on a lake – whatever sounds like heaven to you.

Is there any way you could get a small taste of that feeling this week? An unexpected glimmer you can uncover before you start adulting for the day?

Similar glimmers:
+ *Being surrounded by giant trees ... Perspective.*
+ *Wading into the icy ocean on a hot, still evening.*

Plucking a tomato off the vine

If I were able to make a perfume from anything, it would be the scent of the calyx of a tomato just after it's been picked. Do you know what I'm talking about? If not, go and find out – right now! I'll wait.

The scent is freshness and flavour and surprising hidden depth, all rolled into one. I sniff each calyx that I pluck off tomatoes, and it's an instant glimmer, every time.

Similar glimmers:

+ *Sinking your hand into dry beans (à la* Amélie*).*
+ *Cracking the top of a crème brûlée.*

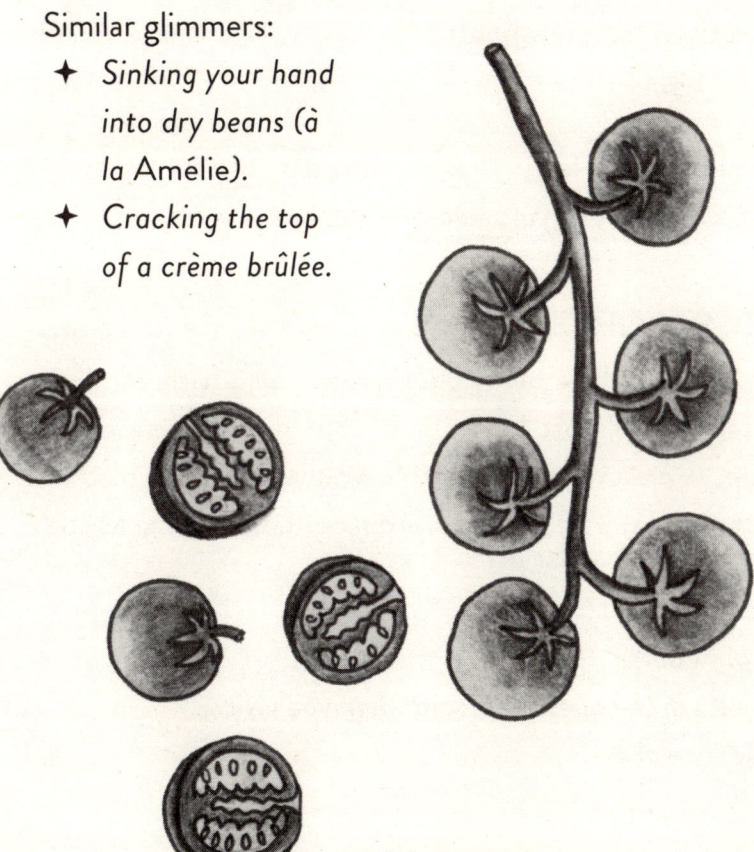

The perfect picnic spot on a hot summer's day

You have all your snacks and drinks, you've got your blanket and they're all starting to feel a little heavy, to be honest. And then you see it – the perfect picnic spot.

Just the right amount of dappled shade, with the sunshine drifting down through the leaves. Contrast is a funny thing, isn't it? In midwinter, all you long for is a patch of warm sunshine, but in summer, a sprinkling of dappled shade becomes a rare and beautiful thing, particularly if you're looking for a picnic spot to relax in for a few hours.

Similar glimmers:
+ *Walking down a leafy, shaded path on a hot day.*
+ *Perfect laundry-drying weather, warm and breezy.*

A framed snapshot

It doesn't have to be a fancy photo, it can be a fairly random pic. In fact, it's almost better if it's random because that's more fun. A picture of people that you love, placed so that you get to look at it all the time, is guaranteed to bring a little hit of joy.

Similar glimmers:
+ *Flowers in the guest bedroom when you visit.*
+ *New shoelaces.*

Killing a mosquito that's been keeping you awake

Have you heard the African proverb: "If you think you're too small to make a difference, you haven't spent the night with a mosquito"? Very true.

Similar glimmers:
+ *Mending a tear in something, so it's as good as new.*
+ *Sharing a skill. Especially if it's something that you can teach easily.*

Free samples or unexpected freebies

I love a good free sample. A little taster at a store, a surprise free sample tucked into an online parcel, a gift-with-purchase I wasn't aware of: I'll take them all. I think it's the allure of surprise – the unexpectedness in a life that is often fairly easy to anticipate.

That's the only problem with being the adult, isn't it? You generally know what the day and week will look like. There's not a whole lot of random surprises to be uncovered. So, if I stumble on a little taste of something delicious, or a teeny sample size of something new, I'm delighted.

Similar glimmers:
+ *An excellent goodie bag at an event.*
+ *A fabulous new outfit (or item of clothing).*

Pizza when the cheese-crust ratio is just right

A good pizza – a great pizza – oh! That is a thing of wonder. Particularly when the cheese to crust ratio is just right, and the crust tastes like something delivered directly from the Dough Gods.

Similar glimmers:

+ *The perfect sourdough, with a caramel crust and a pillowy, soft crumb.*
+ *A slice of watermelon, juice dripping down your chin on a hot summer afternoon.*

Stickers

If you think that adult life doesn't offer too much in the way of delightful silliness, then perhaps it's up to you to sprinkle some delight into the mix?

Stickers are an easy way to do this. Choose some that appeal to you, then stick them in your diary, on shopping lists, on plant pots, in picture frames, inside favourite books and any other spots you can think of – a little moment of silly in the midst of an ordinary day.

Similar glimmers:

+ *Marbles. So pretty! So many colours to choose.*
+ *A carefully placed whoopie cushion. Never gets old.*

Fairy lights (on anything)

I am a sucker for fairy lights. Strung up around the house, in a garden, woven through patio railings and hung in trees. They add a touch of sparkle to anything, and are such a kindness to others who might be walking past and can see them too.

Fairy lights give a kind of soft glow filter to life. What an easy fix!

Similar glimmers:
+ *Googly eyes (on anything, but particularly plant pots).*
+ *Sparklers (on anything, but particularly birthday cake).*

Brown paper packages

A brown paper package may not make you burst into song à la *The Sound of Music*, but there's a good chance it will still give you a little thrill. A wrapped parcel is so intriguing, especially if you're not entirely sure what's in it (or, conversely, if you know exactly what's in it and you're desperate to open it!).

Similar glimmers:
+ *A much-anticipated parcel arriving earlier than expected.*
+ *Balloons. Most kinds, but special mention goes to clear ones with confetti inside, ridiculously shaped foil ones and a bunch of colourful balloons tied on a gate to signal that a party is taking place inside.*

A fabulous fruit salad

There is fruit salad, and then there is fruit salad. A fabulous fruit salad is worth writing home about. It's like a party in your mouth. Mine would include strawberries, mangoes, blueberries and plums. What would you like in yours?

Similar glimmers:
+ *Raspberries (ideally eaten off your fingertips, one by one).*
+ *Biting into a juicy peach (and thinking of* James and the Giant Peach).

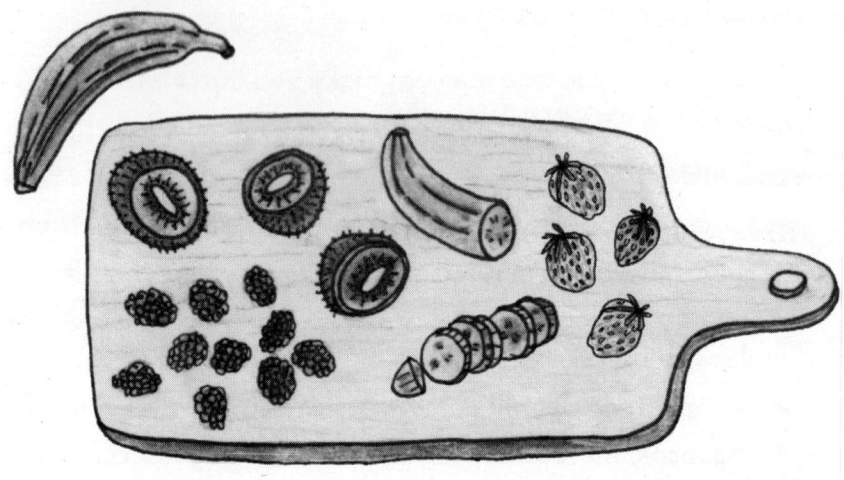

Unnecessary beauty

Unnecessary beauty is everywhere if you train your eyes to see it. Look around you for the small, unnecessary details: frilly metal curlicues on railings, beautiful house numbers, an elaborate pattern of cobblestones, a decorative door handle.

Once your eyes open to unnecessary beauty, you can see it everywhere! It is such a hopeful thing to be on the lookout for; such a testament to the human spirit and the constant quest for creativity.

Similar glimmers:
+ *A wall decal that transforms a dull office space.*
+ *Brightly painted houses.*

Sprinkles (on anything)

Anything looks better with sprinkles on it! It might not *taste* better, but it will look jolly and silly and delightful. I don't mind if they're brightly coloured or metallic, pearls, glimmers or silly shapes, chocolate or teeny tiny candy ... More sprinkles!

Similar glimmers:
+ *Squashing a toasted marshmallow between two cookies.*
+ *Defrosted cake that turns any day into a celebration. (Did you know that you can freeze and defrost cake? And it still tastes great! You're welcome.)*

Sitting outside on the first long summer evening

It seemed impossible for so many months. You almost didn't dare believe this day would come, and now it has ... the evenings are long – properly long. Dusk lingers for what feels like hours, and the air is warm enough to sit outside comfortably without needing layers to keep you warm. It's a promise of all that is to come: relaxation, cold drinks, sunshine and leisure. The first of many long evenings ... What marvellous adventures await?

Similar glimmers:
+ *Eating dinner al fresco.*
+ *Sundowners on a hot day, as the heat lifts and the sun sets.*

Dishwashers

If I were a songwriter, I would write a song about dishwashers – that's how much I love them. It is remarkable to me that you can put dirty dishes into a dishwasher, press a couple of buttons and have gleaming clean dishes emerge a short while later. Truly, I believe it to be one of the most important inventions of the modern age. Instant joy-making!

Similar glimmers:
+ *The ease (and speed) of online shopping.*
+ *The perfect water bottle.*

Rooftop drinks

Any rooftop, any drink. What is it about being on top of a building that feels so exciting? It doesn't matter if it's a cool inner-city bar or your own flat roof – there is something so fun about seeing life from above, saying "Cheers!" to the world.

Similar glimmers:
+ *Coffee and a pastry from a pop-up coffee vendor.*
+ *A chic courtyard café.*

Drawing a face on a piece of fruit

Life can be hard, and boring, and serious. Sometimes all you need is a piece of fruit – orange, banana, anything with a peel really – with a silly face drawn on it to remind you that it's okay to smile. Why not draw a quick face on a piece of fruit in your kitchen right now, either as a surprise for someone else, or a friendly face to greet you when you next walk into the kitchen!

Similar glimmers:
+ *Adding food colouring to banana bread (green banana bread!) or pancakes (blue pancakes!).*
+ *A surprise message or drawing for someone's desk or lunchbox.*

A new pair of pyjamas

It's funny how sometimes you don't invest in the things you use all the time, while the things you use rarely, or that get seen by others, get all the attention. A new pair of pyjamas can feel like such a treat. You could choose anything that you love (whatever picture that conjures up). You're asleep for a third of your life, so you may as well dress up for it!

Similar glimmers:
+ *Beautiful lingerie.*
+ *Soft pillowcases.*

Warm chocolate chip cookies

I'm fairly certain that even if you don't like sweet stuff, a warm chocolate chip cookie will melt your heart. When they've just been taken out of the oven, and the chocolate chips are still melty and gooey, but the cookies itself have firmed up beautifully, and they're practically begging to be accompanied by a lovely cup of tea … Heaven on a plate.

Similar glimmers:
+ *A stack of fresh pancakes.*
+ *Birthday cake. Any kind, really (extra points for sprinkles, of course).*

A wafer cone filled with fresh homemade ice cream

Homemade ice cream or sorbet. Fresh wafer cone. Sunset on a summer's day. What more could anyone ask for?

Similar glimmers:
+ *A slice of ice cream cake (I dare you not to feel like a kid again!).*
+ *A glass of cold milk, chocolate milk or milkshake.*

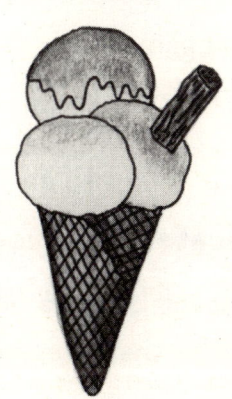

A sincere thank-you card

It doesn't necessarily have to be a card – a message or email will do the trick, too. Someone sincerely thanking you for something you have done is such an unusual delight these days that it's sure to brighten your day.

Similar glimmers:
+ *A handwritten love letter.*
+ *A handmade card or picture.*

Fireworks!

Fireworks in residential areas spook a lot of pets. But organized fireworks over rivers and giant parks, arcing across the sky like magical mythical beasts, are a thing of wonder to behold.

Similar glimmers:
+ *Fireflies!*
+ *Sparklers!*

Delicately scented clothes

The scent is up to you – ocean, lavender, fabric softener. Anything that gives a delicious puff of scent on your clothes.

Similar glimmers:
+ *Soft clothes against your skin.*
+ *Sun-dried sheets.*

A fan on a muggy evening

The air seems to sit, pregnant with heat, unwilling to move. The fan brings a cool gust and rotates away ... and then another cool gust. Whoever invented the electric fan was a genius.

Similar glimmers:
+ *Splashing your face with cold water.*
+ *Putting moisturizer on dry, thirsty, lightly sunburnt skin.*

Anything cooked over an open fire

There is magic in an open fire that makes anything (everything!) taste better. It could be grilled chicken or fish options, but also baked potatoes (almost blackened skin, creamy inside, smoky all the way through) and flatbread (somehow imbued with the fire itself). Even cabbage and lettuce benefit from flame-cooking (smoky, charred, just the right softness). Anything cooked over an open fire seems to transform into the hot, smoky cousin of its usual self.

Similar glimmers:
+ *Homemade chicken soup. So tasty.*
+ *A transformative salad dressing.*

A music festival

Gathered outside in whatever weather summer throws at you, everyone moving to the same beat ... Music festivals have a magic all their own. The organized chaos, the chance to see more than one band perform at once, and the feeling of being released from normal life, even if only for a day or two. Magic.

Similar glimmers:
+ *Coming home from a night out with the songs still playing in your head.*
+ *A heart-wrenching movie that you emerge from, changed.*

A shot of caffeine when you need it

There are few hits as sweet as a shot of caffeine when you really need it, to take you over the finish line (whatever that finish line might be).

I like to ask people what their three favourite "everyday" things are: if you have an unexpected hour off, what would you like to do with that time? A cup of coffee is often mentioned: a simple, everyday treat.

Similar glimmers:
+ *A perfect apple – crunchy, tart and sweet.*
+ *Tea (preferably out of a fine bone china tea cup) and a fresh biscuit.*

Leaning back into the most comfortable chair

"Ahhh ..." A sigh escapes your lips without you noticing. Comfort – specific to you comfort – is a wonderful thing. All the more when it feels as if it was made exactly to your specifications, precisely for this moment, right now.

Similar glimmers:
+ *A snack platter with all the things you like on it, preferably served with a side of friends.*
+ *The ideal office chair: just the right height and bounce for you, specifically.*

A DAILY ROUTINE OF JOY

It's all very well inserting one moment of joy into your everyday life, but is there any way to make your daily routine a little more consistently joyful?

One way is to make a list of five slices of joy from everyday life: nothing difficult to attain, expensive or complicated; just five simple things. Then make a list of five things you do every day and compare the two. Could you add or subtract anything to help them match up better? Join the dots between something you love doing and something you have to do?

I am inspired by Virginia Woolf, who said, "Every season is likeable, and wet days and fine, red wine and white, company and solitude."[18] There are small joys to be found in most circumstances if you're willing to look for them.

You don't have to wait around for The Next Big Thing: a daily life of small joys is more than enough.

"The great revelation perhaps never did come," Woolf wrote. "Instead, there were little daily miracles, illuminations, matches struck unexpectedly in the dark; here was one."[19]

Have there been any little daily miracles you've noticed this week?

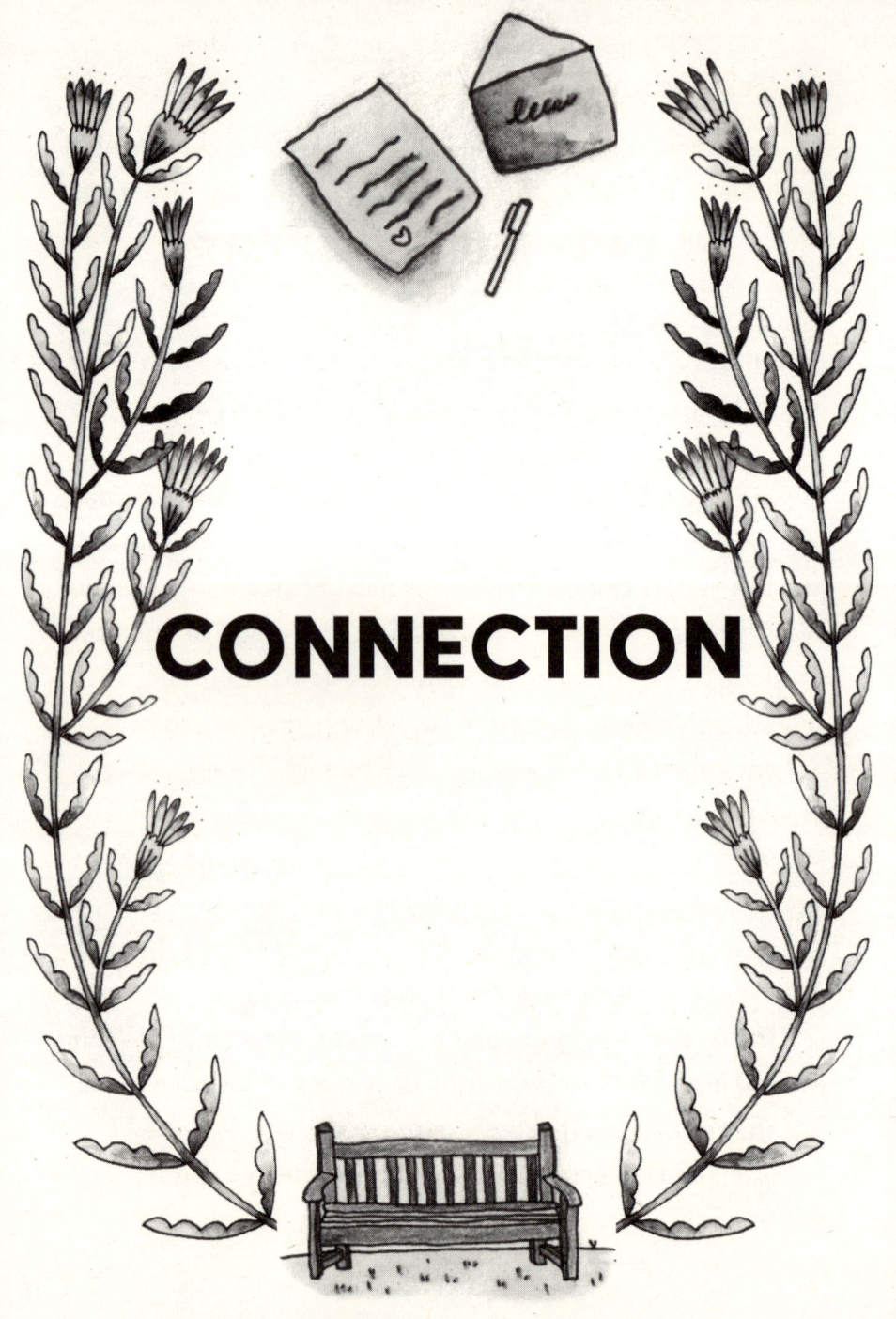

CONNECTION

Understanding love languages

Do you know about the languages of love? They are an enormously helpful tool to figure out how you give love and, crucially, how you want to receive it. There are five "love languages", as conceived by Gary Chapman in *The Five Love Languages*. They are:

1. Words of affirmation (written or spoken)
2. Acts of service (chores)
3. Receiving gifts (bought, made or found)
4. Quality time
5. Physical touch[20]

Most people like all of them but favour one or two. To make it interesting, the one you give is not always the same as the one you want to receive. Do you know which one is your love language? What about your family/friends/partner's?

Once you work out someone's love language, you can ensure you're speaking it so that they truly feel loved. And once you work out your own, you can tell your loved ones how to show you that they care.

Similar glimmers:
+ *Totally understanding what someone is trying to explain. "Am I making sense?" they ask. "Yes! I totally get it."*
+ *A sincere, "I love you".*

A surprise snack after work

You're on your way out after work, meeting your partner or friend, and they bring you a little snack in case you're feeling a bit peckish. What a beautiful expression of love.

Similar glimmers:
+ *Someone baking a cake for tea, and inviting you over.*
+ *Cousins that are like friends (but even better).*

Feeling part of a community

Feeling part of a community has been shown to promote greater resilience, reduce depression and anxiety, and help you feel part of something bigger than yourself.

Can you find a way to feel part of a community? It can be a physical thing, in your neighbourhood or at your workplace, or online. It really is a special feeling to be plugged into people who understand you.

Similar glimmers:
+ *Helping someone. It is particularly satisfying to fill a need that doesn't ask a lot of you but makes a big difference to the other person (lifting something heavy, decoding something tech-related, explaining something that is simple to you, but not to others).*
+ *Taking a home-made meal to new parents.*

Total agreement

You know that feeling when you totally agree with someone about something you thought was unique to you? It's as if the door to your mind opened up a chink, and found an equal and opposite chink in the person sitting across from you. "You too?! I thought it was just me!"

Similar glimmers:
+ *Feeling supported. Maybe it's practical support – a meal or a ride somewhere. Maybe it's physical support – a hug at just the right moment. Maybe it's emotional support – a call or message when you need it.*
+ *A true friendship, one where you can let all your truths hang out, and still be accepted.*

A fire ritual

Have you ever been to a fire ritual? It is a beautiful thing. People gathered around a large fire, offering something into the flames, and standing together in meditative silence as whatever they are letting go of gets burnt to ashes. Magic.

Similar glimmers:
+ *Watching a bonfire blaze (the awe, tinged with a little fear).*
+ *Making space for meaning in the busyness of modern life.*

"No need to reply."

One of the things I found most difficult when my dad was very ill in hospital was having to update people. Putting my feelings into words made it worse, because I couldn't ignore how awful things were.

One day a friend checked in on me and ended her message with these four beautiful words: *No need to reply.* The relief washed over me. One less thing to do! One less person to report back to. Now I use these words all the time, whenever I want to send someone love but don't want to pressure them into responding.

Similar glimmers:
+ *"See how you feel."*
+ *"No rush."*

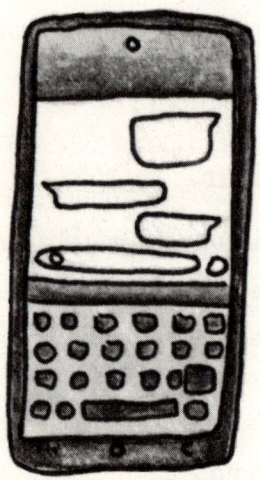

Reconnecting with an old friend

The older I get, the more I understand that sometimes a friendship is about timing more than personality. You reconnect and some critical aspect of your life has changed and boom! The time is right. What luck that you connected with each other again.

Similar glimmers:

+ *Connecting with someone over a shared passion for a TV show.*
+ *Casual, meandering chats.*

Made-up family holidays

What do you and your family love doing most? Whether it's your actual family or friends, why not make up a new family holiday? For example, in my family we have an Annual Pasta Day. Once a year, my children get to eat buttery pasta for breakfast, lunch and dinner, because my children love pasta more than anything else. What could this be for you?

Similar glimmers:

+ *Take a young person out for a treat, like a parent-child date night, but for any child in your life.*
+ *A daily dinner ritual (like lighting a candle or sharing "one good thing that happened today").*

Really listening

True listening is rare. No interruptions, no advice-giving, no telling of a reciprocal story ... Just listening. Perhaps the occasional nod or grunt of acknowledgement. An invitation to, "Say more about that?" Giving that kind of attention is delicious.

Similar glimmers:
+ *Really being listened to.*
+ *Walking naturally in step with someone.*

Appreciating the partner of a friend

On some level, it makes sense to assume that if you really like your friend, you will naturally like the person they choose as a partner. But live through enough awkward interactions with friends' partners and you'll know that is not always the case. So, when the stars align and it turns out that you not only really like your friend (naturally) but also truly enjoy their partner, well! That is something to celebrate.

Similar glimmers:
+ *Games Night. Particularly with fun friends and lots of laughter.*
+ *A weekly friend ritual (Wednesday movie nights, Thursday coffees, Friday walks, etc.).*

"You made my day!"

When your day can be made by the teeniest slice of joy, you can offer the gift of, "You made my day!" to someone. This can be someone helping you out unexpectedly at work, or fixing something you didn't think could be mended, or even just holding the elevator door for you when you're running late. The goal is a low bar for delight, and this one works as a glimmer for both of you. Want to give it a try?

Similar glimmers:
+ *"You go first."*
+ *"I made you a cup of tea."*

A phone call that goes on so long you have to pee

The joy of a phone call with someone you love. You think it'll just be a quick chat, but then it turns out you both have so much to say! And you're enjoying the conversation so much, it flows and flows until you suddenly realize how long you've been chatting because you desperately need to pee. The best.

Similar glimmers:
+ *Leaning against a bridge, watching the lights reflect in the water, chatting.*
+ *Lingering outside a restaurant because you have so much to talk about but it's actually time to go home.*

A shared joke

You start telling the story and before you're even halfway in, the other person is already snorting with laughter because they remember, they were there. Shared memories, shared jokes. Absolute gold.

Similar glimmers:
+ *Telling a funny story and making everyone laugh.*
+ *Both of you finding the same thing hilarious.*

The spaces between

When visitors come to stay, it's often the headline events that get the attention – going out for a lovely meal or a big celebration, that kind of thing. But I'm convinced it's the in-between moments that really matter. The moments when you're hanging around the kitchen counter, chopping vegetables, or clearing the table, or drinking a morning cuppa in your pyjamas before you get ready to start the day. The beautiful ordinary stuff: that's where the magic lies.

Similar glimmers:
+ *Sharing life stories.*
+ *"You are doing so well." There's something magical about these five words because so often it feels as if the effort you're making is going unnoticed. And then someone notices! And recognizes your effort. What a gift.*

A hug so tight you know you're loved

Some people give the best hugs. They walk up to you, fold you in their arms and you can feel the love radiating through them. All your cares seem to dissolve for a moment. You feel safe, and warm, and loved.

Similar glimmers:
+ *A morning cuddle.*
+ *Stroking someone's back.*

An excellent toast

A good toast is difficult – they are often boring, too long and inexpertly delivered. The bar is so low that it feels almost euphoric to listen to an excellent one. Cheers to that!

Similar glimmers:
+ *Catching a joke and building on it.*
+ *A genuine laugh-out-loud joke.*

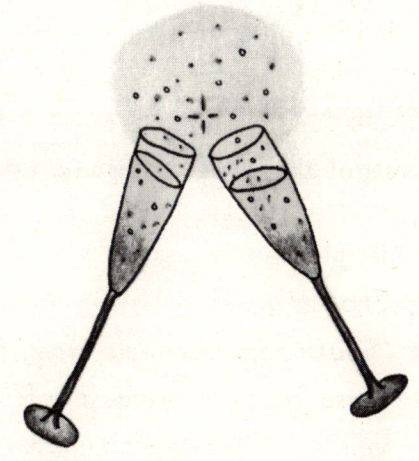

A surprise, sincere compliment

I know very few people who can comfortably accept a compliment, without attempting to brush it off or pretend it's not true. Why is that?

When I was thirteen, I went away on a school camp and one of the modules was about how to accept a compliment. Their advice was that, instead of simply saying, "Thank you", you should say, "Please elaborate!"

Try it out! I guarantee that if nothing else, it will make the other person laugh in disbelief.

Similar glimmers:
+ *Speaking to like-minded souls.*
+ *When you hear: "Thank you for doing that for me." Especially lovely when you thought whatever you were doing went unnoticed.*

Being treated to a meal

"I've got this one!" they say, taking the bill from the table. Yay! What a treat.

Similar glimmers:
+ *Treating someone to a meal.*
+ *Ordering delicious food to be delivered to someone.*

The snigger of recognition

It's not an outright laugh, not an exclamation of, "Yes! Me too!" The snigger of recognition is its quieter sister: very revealing if you can catch it before it disappears.

Similar glimmers:
+ *A running joke.*
+ *A catchphrase that somehow applies to everything for a few days (usually while away on holiday, and often never again).*

Sideways listening

Sideways listening is my favourite because it's the kind of listening that feels comfortable to everyone. Instead of sitting across from someone and looking them in the eye, you listen while walking, driving or preparing dinner together. It's listening under the guise of some other activity that doesn't take up any of your brainpower. And it opens the doorway to conversations that are often more frank and honest.

Similar glimmers:
+ *Sense-checking your thinking about something with someone you trust.*
+ *Not needing to fill every silence to feel comfortable: companionable silence.*

Being understood

This might be what everyone is looking for in life. Just to be understood. For someone to look at you and say: "I see you, as you are. And it is good."

Similar glimmers:
+ *Feeling safe enough to be vulnerable.*
+ *Being seen in your best light: your actions being interpreted generously and kindly.*

The connection of strangers

You've all been waiting in the airport together, then on the same small plane for how many hours? Nobody even remembers. Then queuing to get off, and get your bags and finally disperse, never to see each other again.

But in those hours you share, there's a kind of grace and kindness you extend to each other, all living through an almost identical experience. It's unusual, in our mostly-solitary lives, and quite lovely.

Similar glimmers:
+ *The eye roll you share with other commuters when it's announced that the train is delayed.*
+ *The shared relief when you've been waiting at a bus stop together for ages, and the bus finally comes into sight.*

Being told a story

I don't really care if it's an ancient Irish myth, the story of what happened to you when you were five, or the big drama at work today. I love a good story – being invited into a different world, with a whole cast of characters and a plot line I can't yet anticipate.

Similar glimmers:
+ *When people use old-fashioned words naturally in conversation: "Jeepers!" or "Crikey!"*
+ *Listening to someone with a wonderful vocabulary describe something.*

Someone helping you look for something

"I can't find my ... !" you exclaim, frustrated. "It was just here! I could have sworn I put it there!"

And then, if it's something important, that sense of cold dread that you haven't only lost it but Lost It, and it will never be found again. Someone else willingly entering into this mess is a real gift. And a real balm to the fear, because surely two sets of eyes are better than one?

Similar glimmers:
+ *Remembering someone's birthday.*
+ *Someone doing you a favour.*

Rituals (any type or tradition)

Some people grow up in houses steeped in tradition: religious and specific holiday celebrations, family dinners and deeply entrenched ways to mark time passing. Other people, not so much. But as an adult, you get to choose what rituals you want to create, what traditions you want to build on to or create from the ground up.

Whether it's linked to religion or the calendar, a celebration or the passing of time, marked with song or food, fire or the full moon, there is something profound about an intentional ritual.

Similar glimmers:
+ *A poem that feels like it was written for you.*
+ *A guided meditation that really resonates.*

"How was your day?" (Really)

Casual, social interactions are an important part of the fabric of society. But often there's not a lot of space to unpack an answer to a casual greeting. There is a time and place for that kind of interaction, of course, but there is also a time and place for someone authentically wanting to know how you are, how your day was, what happened, and how you feel about it. And then giving you all the time you need to unpack it as slowly as necessary.

Similar glimmers:
+ *An authentic, "How are things going at work?"*
+ *A text asking, "How was your week?" from someone who really cares.*

A surprise party (that actually works)

Most surprise parties don't quite work, let's be honest – someone tells, or the person guesses, or it falls flat because they're already in their pyjamas and don't open the door ... Which is why it's such a treat when a surprise party actually works! And the person is delighted! Flabbergasted, even.

Similar glimmers:
+ *Celebrating the wedding of two friends.*
+ *A birthday party invitation (for someone you really like).*

A gift that shows how well someone knows you

This is a pretty enormous slice of joy for me. Any gift is lovely, of course, but when someone goes out on a limb and gives you a present they're sure you'll like, it says a lot. When they get it right, and the gift is so perfectly "you" that you couldn't have chosen it better yourself, well. That's a special feeling.

Similar glimmers:
+ *A heartfelt card.*
+ *A little love note.*

Overflowing conversations

You have so much to talk about, you don't know where to begin! And then once you do begin, you have to cross your fingers so you can remember what you wanted to say without interrupting. And then circle back to the thing you were talking about before, because actually, you agree!

I always think of these conversations as pots filled with brightly coloured ingredients, all popping up to the surface because the pot is boiling so rapidly.

Similar glimmers:
+ *Dinner party conversation that excites the mind.*
+ *A conversation that sparks something in you that you can't stop thinking about.*

"I never thought of that before!"

Few phrases make me feel more like a genius than being told, "I never thought of that before!" Next time someone surprises you with a fresh idea, let them know!

Sharing and receiving appreciation shows the conversation has spark and vibrancy, and that there are good ingredients in here, not just the same old ideas being rehashed. Can you offer the gift of, "I never thought of that before" to someone today?

Similar glimmers:
+ *Giving someone space to find a solution to their problem all by themselves.*
+ *Not judging someone's behaviour too soon, so that they can talk it through.*

FINDING FUN

Sometimes life seems to grind you down, doesn't it? The meetings, the family obligations, the deadlines ... Your tasks suck all the colour out of every day. At times like these, it may be necessary to actively look for things that are fun, frivolous and light-hearted. Unsurprisingly, this might be hard to do.

✦ A new definition of "fun"

Fun, according to the dictionary, is:

1. a source of enjoyment, amusement, diversion
2. pleasure, gaiety, or merriment
3. jest or sport[21]

Gosh, that feels hard to attain. Amusement! Gaiety! Merriment! Jest! Yikes. But perhaps your version of fun has different words attached to it? Nobody said you can't write your own definition.

I think fun changes as you get older. What you used to call fun – drinking, staying up late, hordes of strangers

– might not appeal in the same way. So, what's fun for you, right now?

✦ Gentle kinds of fun

Every so often a music festival or a night out dancing is fantastic, but if I think about what I've really enjoyed in the last few months, it's a gentle kind of fun. A tea party with all my brothers and our kids crowded around a delicious cake. A fancy dinner out with friends where we all dressed up. A silly movie at the cinema with girlfriends.

Artist Keeley Shaw's words struck a chord with me: "I hope you find fun again – maybe not the extravagant, bubbling, larger than life kind – but the simple, quiet kind – I hope you find fun in the glow of candle light – in walks to nowhere in particular – in long conversations that leave you smiling."[22]

I think there's a definition of fun that is more like a burbling brook than a waterfall. It doesn't leave you gasping for air, but fills you up gently and sustainably. It's found in long talks with friends, lazy lunches, not hurrying, and saying no to things unless you really (really!) want to say yes.

✦ More laughter

One direct route to fun is laughing more. But it won't necessarily happen on its own – you have to invite laughter in.

Go to live comedy shows, watch funny shows on TV, choose light-hearted books rather than only books rooted in reality. One foolproof tactic for me is a monthly Games Night where three couples get together and play a silly board game. It's not about being competitive, it's just about having a break from the daily drudge. Perhaps instead of fixating on the word fun, the goal should be things that make you laugh?

✦ Be spontaneous

My suggestion, as you look for more fun, is to throw a bit of randomness into the hunt. A bit of spontaneity and unpredictability. Even if the actual thing you do isn't particularly fun, the fact that you're doing it at an odd time of day might be. For example, instead of going for a morning walk, take a stroll at sunset. Instead of eating lunch at your desk, walk outside and eat it in the sunshine, or – better yet – meet a friend for a quick lunch. If you're usually watching TV on the couch by 8pm each evening, take yourself to an 8pm movie at the cinema instead. Mix up the routine a little.

The spontaneity can be tiny, too. You could switch up what you listen to on the way to work: instead of a podcast or the news, listen to your favourite album from when you were 21. Play classical music while you make your breakfast. Wear brightly coloured socks that nobody has to see. It only takes a fissure to let the light in.

The idea isn't to create vast and scary change, but to remind yourself that there are opportunities for surprise and delight in even the tightest schedule.

✦ Spend your pocket money

Have you heard the phrase, "Adults are just tall kids with lots of pocket money"? It's easy to forget what it feels like to be excited about small things. Is there something small and fun you could spend a little bit of money on? If you did have pocket money, where would it go? Essentially: how could you treat yourself?

✦ Little things, big impact

My husband's granny collected beautiful blue-and-white striped crockery, and only ever used it for special occasions. She gave it to her son, who saved it for special occasions. They gave it to us, and we now use it every day. And yes, there are a few chips and the occasional breakage, but they bring us daily joy.

What I'm saying is: use all the lovely notebooks you've been saving up. Light all the scented candles. Buy yourself flowers if they bring you a little burst of joy. Wear the lovely jacket. Do the little things that make your heart warm. Whatever breaks you out of the humdrum of daily life is worth it.

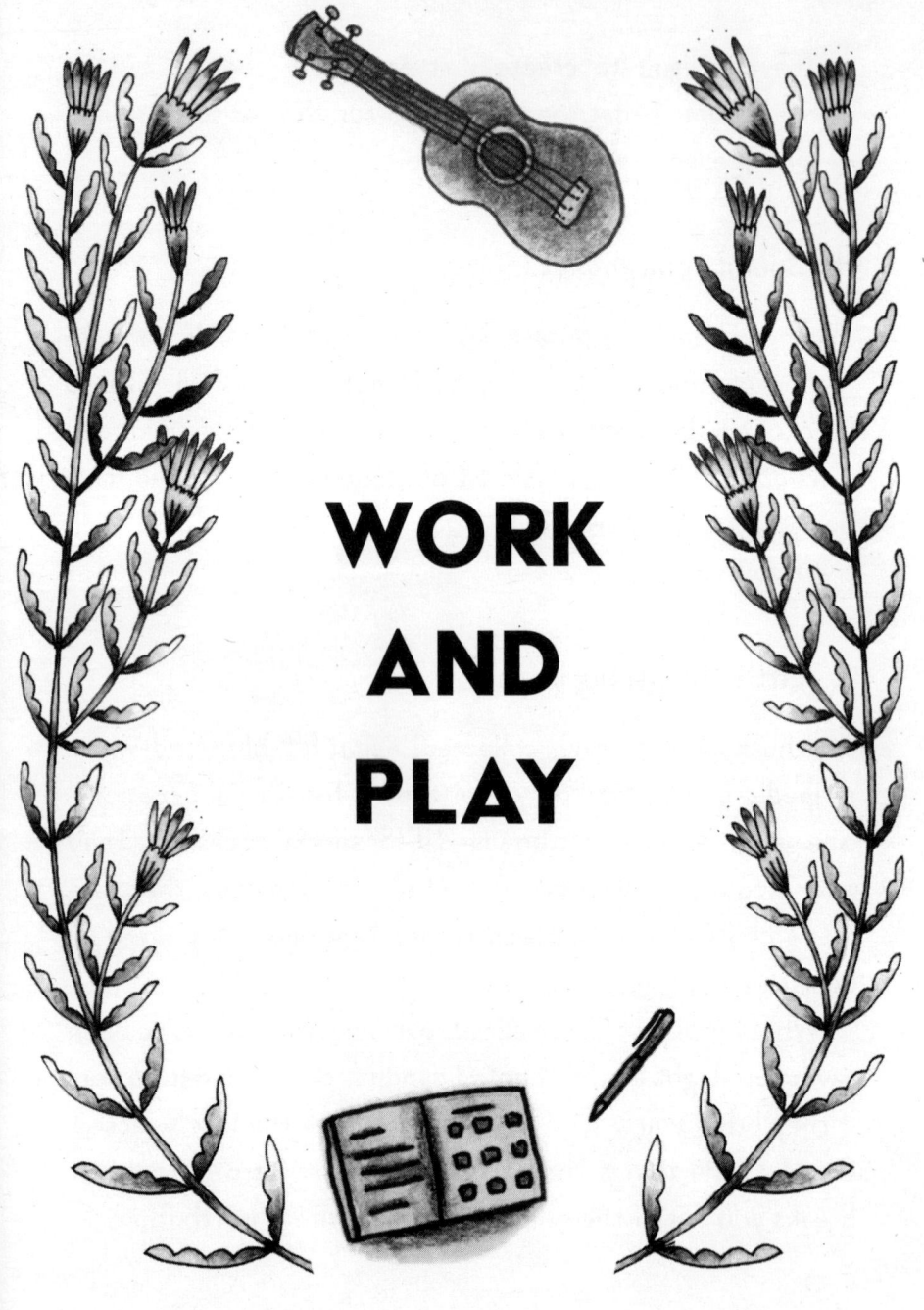

WORK
AND
PLAY

Waking up early to work

I love a lie-in. I love a natural wake-up. But I also, conversely, love waking up super-early while the rest of the house sleeps, quietly making myself a cup of tea, switching on my desk lamp and getting stuck into a chunky work project. It has to be chunky or I wouldn't sacrifice sleep, but there is magic in the early morning that makes it feel as if time unspools at a slower pace.

It's not a card I can play often, or it loses its magic, but when I do play it I get a certain thrill that the magic still works.

Similar glimmers:
+ *Looking for the exact right word, and finding it.*
+ *A few hours of productive work.*

Birthday cake in the office

Most adults become five-years-old again when a birthday cake emerges in an office. Eating cake in the middle of a work day, and maybe even singing "Happy Birthday", is a brief reprieve from adult life.

Similar glimmers:
+ *Office snacks that somehow taste better than they do at home.*
+ *A really excellent work lunch with colleagues.*

Meeting an online colleague in real life

Hybrid and remote working have a lot of perks, but one of the deeply strange things about not going into an office is that you can work with someone for months before finding out if they are really as tall as you imagine.

A real slice of joy is meeting someone in person for the first time and truly connecting. You knew you liked each other from your online interactions, but you *actually* like each other in real life. What a win!

Similar glimmers:
+ *Casual chit-chat with your colleagues as you make coffee.*
+ *Connecting with a colleague over a shared interest that has nothing to do with work.*

Friday late afternoon

You've finally reached the point where people have stopped playing email ping-pong and replying to your emails as quickly as you send them. Thank heavens.

Similar glimmers:
+ *Shutting down your computer for the weekend.*
+ *Writing your Out of Office auto-responder before a much-anticipated break.*

A shared (niche) passion

Perhaps the greatest gift of a job you love is that you can nerd out about whatever your niche expertise is. And you'll be in good company. Whether it's growing flowers, molecular gastronomy or complicated database management, you'll have others who share your passion. You have found your place, and can tend to it lovingly.

Similar glimmers:
+ *A job well done.*
+ *Appreciating someone else's niche knowledge.*

The giddiness of the last day of work (or school)

No matter how much you love your work (and I really hope you do), the last day of work, school or college for the year is a thrilling one. It can be before you go on summer or Christmas holidays, the countdown to a much-anticipated trip, taking a few days off at the end of a project, wrapping up the tax year, or whatever "the year" means for you. The rest of the To Do List will have to wait. You've done your best, and now it's time to Officially Unwind.

Similar glimmers:
+ *Taking a sick day without any work repercussions.*
+ *Booking a random afternoon off, just because you can.*

Exercise buddies

One of the joys of exercising with other people is the casual, laughter-filled complaints that inevitably ensue when the teacher asks you to do something difficult. There is such camaraderie there, such shared experience, even if it's only for one hour a week.

Similar glimmers:
+ *Finding exercise you truly enjoy doing.*
+ *The ideal exercise teacher for you.*

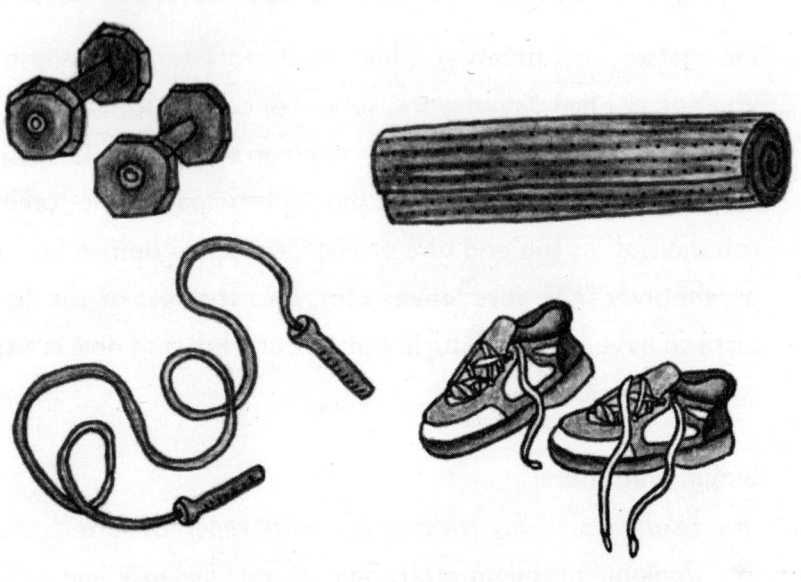

Waving at the end of video calls

Adults are not often adorable. But the way pretty much everyone – routinely, regularly, as a matter of course – waves at the end of video calls is actually adorable, if you think about it. Nobody is shy about it, or rolls their eyes. Everyone merrily waves like school kids leaving the school gates.

Similar glimmers:
+ *Hair looking good on a video call.*
+ *Appreciating in-person workshops because they seemed impossible for so long.*

Flexible working

It's like the whole world has woken up to the fact that employees have homes, families and lives outside of work. And while some jobs are back full-time, others have taken a more flexible, lenient approach. There's a whole bouquet of benefits: it's easier for parents, reduces commuting time, saves money and improves work-life balance. Whether it's only a nod to a flexible working life, or a wholehearted embrace, at least this lingo is now part of our daily work lexicon.

Similar glimmers:
+ *Inbox zero!*
+ *Moments of work-life balance, no matter how brief.*

Asking for help, and getting it

It's not always easy asking for help, particularly in a work context. So, when you can gather your courage and ask for help from someone who can legitimately make things easier, and they do, well! What a relief.

Similar glimmers:
+ *A meeting of minds.*
+ *A shared lived experience: when you both speak the same language about a certain issue because you live with it every day.*

Time to think

Being given time to think is such a gift. As in, time to think, and also Time To Think, the thinking environment created by Nancy Kline.[23] It is a very practical approach to work (and life) that involves listening deeply and not interrupting, so that people can do their best thinking. The difference is palpable. It's like being taken from a busy city street to a cool, shady garden: an opportunity for your mind to exhale.

Similar glimmers:
+ *A snowball of an idea that starts with a core thought that other people add to and you keep building it together.*
+ *Feeling heard. Seen. Acknowledged.*

The ideal amount of procrastination

There's procrastination, and *procrastination*. I'm talking about creative procrastination that takes your mind on a meander to unexpected places. When you find that sweet spot of procrastination – perhaps a little time spent outdoors, a movie trailer, some joy spotting online – it can act as fertilizer for whatever idea you're trying to grow.

The truth is that you're not a productivity monkey, primed to work all day. Everyone has their own specific rhythm, and sometimes procrastination can help you find yours.

Similar glimmers:
+ *Hitting the magical state of flow while you're working.*
+ *Needing less time than you thought to complete a task.*

When hard work is recognized

Much of adult life can feel like slaving away without anyone noticing. But then sometimes, someone recognizes how hard you've been working. They call it out, and shine it up, and reflect it back to you. The feedback is specific and personal. You are seen, you are appreciated. It was worth it.

Similar glimmers:
+ *A pen that writes beautifully.*
+ *Getting more money than expected back on your tax return.*

An enthusiastic meeting

So many meetings are perfunctory or a little boring. But every so often you chance upon the unicorn of meetings: everyone is enthusiastic, the subject matter is valid and important, and it feels as if actual decisions have been made that will effect change. It's like paddling a canoe with your hands, and then suddenly being given an oar.

Similar glimmers:
+ *Workshopping that works (unusual, but beautiful).*
+ *That lightbulb feeling when you solve a problem.*

"Eating the ugly frog" first

You look at your To Do List for the day, and tackle the hardest task before you do anything else. The hardest task might be difficult in terms of complexity, or mental labour required, or it might be something you don't want to do (make a phone call, in my case!).

Whatever it is that you're putting off, do that thing first. The rest of the day, no matter what it throws at you, will feel easier because you dealt with that ugly frog first.

Similar glimmers:
+ *Resisting the lure of procrastination.*
+ *Feeling fired up to "get shit done".*

Finding a new hobby

Finding a new hobby is like uncovering a treasure box in your own back garden – so unexpected! So delightful! Whether it's a sport or a craft, a passion for a specific type of cooking or a love of complicated machinery, a hobby can add a brilliant touch of zest to any day.

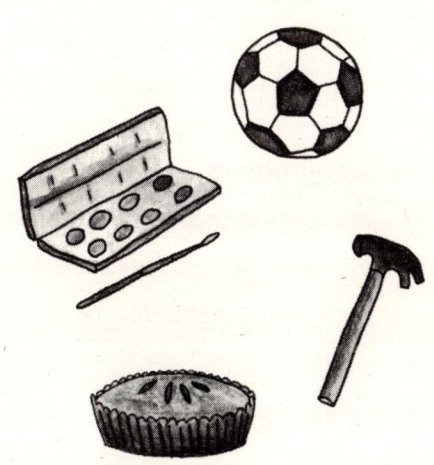

Similar glimmers:

+ *Discovering a new TV show that you absolutely love.*
+ *A new snack that you can't get enough of.*

Starting the week refreshed

It doesn't always happen. But on those Mondays when you wake up and feel refreshed by your weekend, rested and ready to tackle whatever the week throws at you, it's as if all the stars have aligned in your favour.

Similar glimmers:

+ *A day when everything seems to go your way.*
+ *Nailing it. Whatever "it" is.*

Being eloquent in a meeting

You have something to say. You're not entirely sure how to say it. You reach for the words and ... they come! You find exactly the right words to encapsulate precisely what it is you want to communicate. It doesn't happen every time, but when it does, it feels like getting to the top of a mountain, with a spectacular view laid out in front of you.

Similar glimmers:
+ *A meeting that resolves something.*
+ *Writing a three-line email that succinctly says everything necessary.*

A meeting cancelled on a busy day

Your day looks intense. You feel as if you're at the starting line of a marathon, and while you know you *can* do it (because you have to), there's no sense of positive anticipation about the amount of energy required.

And then! Out of nowhere, a meeting gets cancelled. A window of opportunity opens up, and with it, a fresh breeze. What sweet, sweet relief!

Similar glimmers:
+ *A moment of rest in a busy day.*
+ *Finishing a meeting early.*

Casual but friendly social encounters

It's so easy to get caught up in labelling people. These are my Close Friends. These are my Work Colleagues. These are Acquaintances. This is the Coffee Guy. But if you think about it, those casual but friendly social encounters knit together the fabric of society.

Perhaps all you say to each other is, "How are you? Good! Have a nice day." But interactions like these connect your days in ways that can be hard to see until they're gone.

What if you imbued every casual but friendly social encounter this week with a little more intent, an extra ray of sunshine? What might that look like?

Similar glimmers:
- *Reconnecting with an acquaintance you really like.*
- *A walk-and-talk with someone you haven't seen in a while.*

Purposefully firing off emails

It's almost as if your fingers have a mind of their own, flying across the keyboard and dispatching email after email. The thrill of productivity when you step into the flow is sublime.

Similar glimmers:
- *A sense of empowerment.*
- *That "just stepped out of a salon" feeling.*

Work besties

It may only happen once. It may never happen at all. But if you are lucky enough to find a work friend, consider yourself deeply blessed. Someone who you authentically enjoy spending time with, and would happily hang out with every day even if you weren't being paid! What luck.

Similar glimmers:
+ *A pleasant office environment.*
+ *A lovely view from your desk.*

Getting stronger (mentally or physically)

Getting stronger is immensely empowering – whether it's physical or mental – particularly as you age. It's easy to imagine you'll always be young and able to master any new concept that is thrown your way. To recognize a weakness and then get stronger in that area is a vital and empowering feeling. For me, it was learning about financial management. It could also be lifting weights, running, getting therapy, learning to code – anything that you feel is holding you back from being your strongest self.

Similar glimmers:
+ *Doing something you didn't think you could do.*
+ *Mastering a new recipe.*

Handling conflict well

Conflict in the workplace is even more sticky because you still have to work together tomorrow, and the next day, and the day after that. So when there's a conflict situation that you manage to handle well, that is cause for celebration.

I always remember what a colleague said to me after we had resolved some conflict: "Where there's no rain, it's a desert." Relationships are not supposed to be sunshine all the time – a little rain (a little conflict) can be helpful to clear the air.

Similar glimmers:
+ *Doing something creative around people who 100 per cent believe you can do it.*
+ *An adult discussion about a difficult topic.*

Finishing a project knowing you did your best

There are many things you don't have control over, but you control how much effort you put into them. Did you show up as your whole self for this project and give it your all? There is satisfaction in knowing you could not have done any better.

Similar glimmers:
+ *A knotty problem that suddenly untangles itself (often when you stop trying so damn hard).*
+ *Completing something you've been putting off.*

Unplugging from devices for a day

It almost seems impossible to unplug from all your devices for a day, doesn't it? Computer, phone, social media, the works! But it is possible. And when you do, your sense of time recalibrates. It's no longer about reaching for your phone to check your messages or being dragged back to your notifications to see the comments on your latest post.

Time recalibrates to: Now. And the now after that. Even if it's only for one day, the mental rest and relaxation from no devices is like a hot tub for the mind.

Similar glimmers:
+ *So few emails you wonder if there's something wrong with your internet (rare but precious).*
+ *A day of no meetings.*

A good idea

Every so often an idea comes along that gets you excited. It might present itself when you are least expecting it. When you share it with someone else, the excitement builds. It is a good idea! They agree! Zing!

Similar glimmers:
+ *Listening to a talk that changes the way you think.*
+ *Learning a new skill that helps you do your job better.*

Choosing rest

Did you know that there are seven different types of rest?

1. **Physical rest:** either passive (sleep) or active (stretching, yoga, massage).
2. **Mental rest:** slowing down the hamster wheel of thoughts.
3. **Sensory rest:** escaping from the over-stimulation of too much going on.
4. **Creative rest:** turning to nature and the arts for inspiration.
5. **Emotional rest:** time and space to express all your feelings.
6. **Social rest:** prioritizing the relationships that energize you.
7. **Spiritual rest:** focusing on something greater than yourself.

Choosing rest can seem like a radical act, given how obsessed the world is with productivity. Why not try it this week?

Similar glimmers:
+ *Speaking up for yourself.*
+ *Prioritizing self-care.*

Birdsong while you work

It can be hard to focus on small things when there are Big Things to be considered. Is this the right job? Do you know what you're doing? Are you following your purpose?

But it is helpful to draw the lens all the way back, and recognize the beauty of the tiny. Can you hear any birds while you work? Does the light slant through the window in a particularly lovely way? Is there a pleasant scent in the air? All those little glimmers count, too. They add meaning.

Similar glimmers:
+ *A slow weekday morning to ease into the day.*
+ *An uninterrupted afternoon to work.*

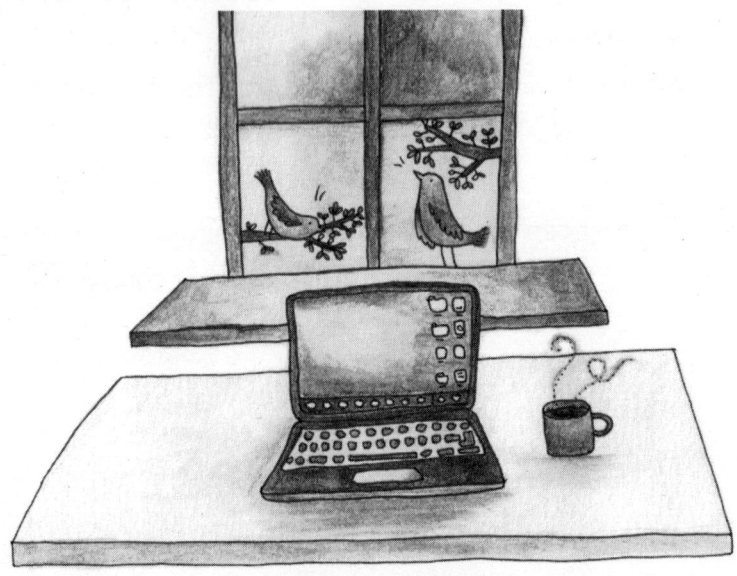

Committing to a new habit

You've heard it takes 21 days to start forming a new habit, but you're not *entirely* sure you want to commit. It's a revelation when you decide you do, actually, want to change something or start something new, and you will, actually, commit to it. It can be as simple as drinking a certain amount of water every day, taking the stairs instead of the elevator or reading a daily glimmer every morning. Or it could be as complex as learning a new language. Whatever it is, you've committed now. Watch this space, world! New things await!

Similar glimmers:

✦ *Changing your cushion covers or the handles on the kitchen cupboards (or some other minor but dramatic decor change).*

✦ *Clearing out a space in your home that's been cluttered for years.*

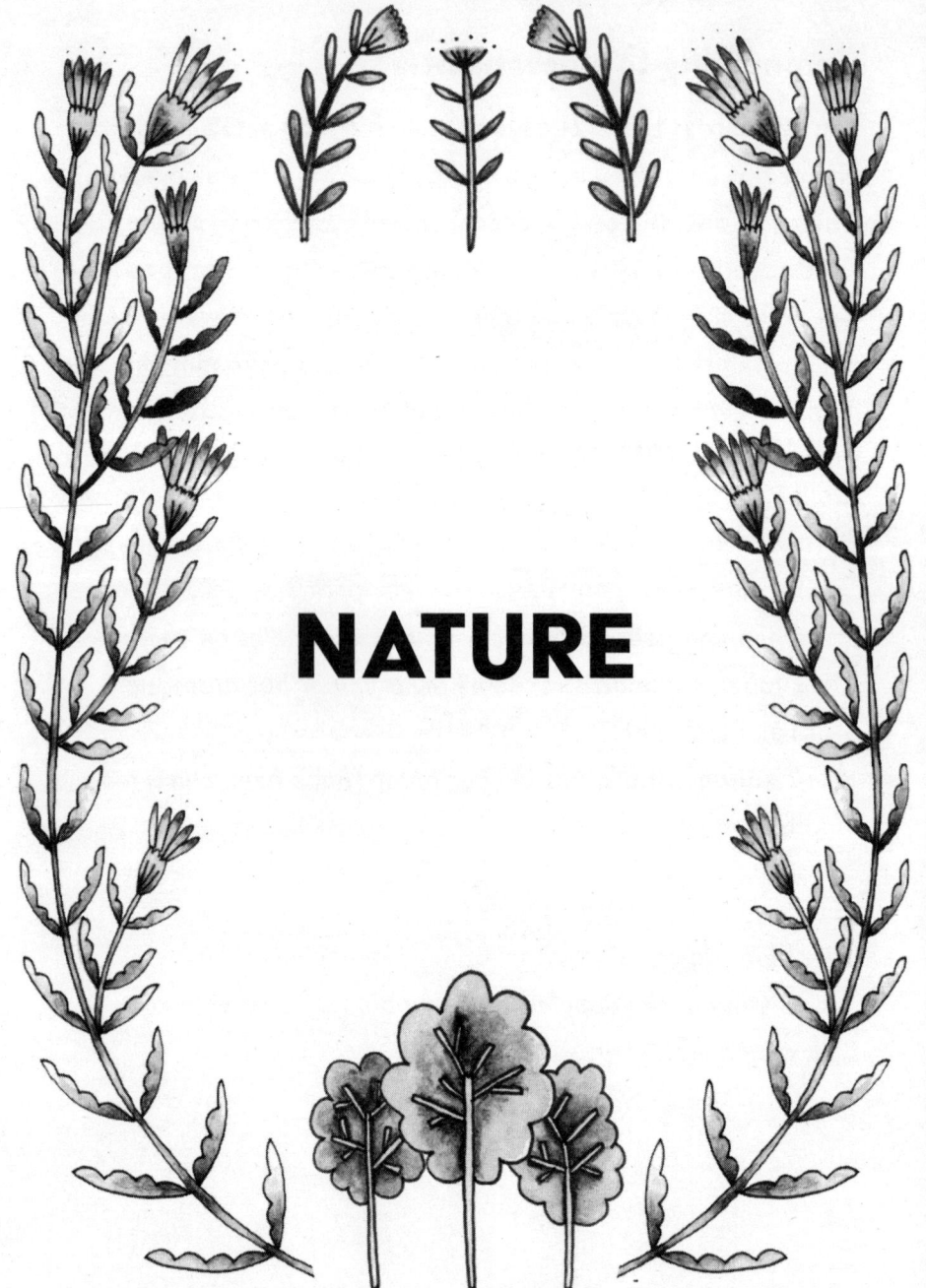

NATURE

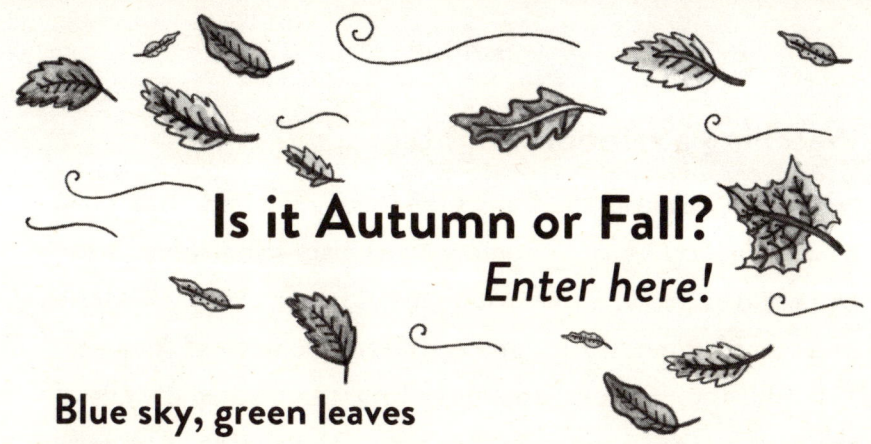

Is it Autumn or Fall?
Enter here!

Blue sky, green leaves

Studies have shown that being outside and looking up at trees and the sky while listening to birdsong is good for mental wellbeing.[24] I feel like you could have figured this one out without a study, but maybe we all need reminding?

Gazing upward, through green leaves, at a blue sky is deeply calming. The colours seem to signal to the nervous system that you can exhale and relax ... It's time to unwind.

Even if all you do is grab five minutes of outside time, staring up at the sky, it can have a profound impact on how you feel when you head back indoors. Studies have shown!

Similar glimmers:
+ *Floating on an inflatable: blue sky above, endlessly.*
+ *Sitting in the dappled shade by a river (preferably on a picnic blanket, with a book).*

Watching a rainbow brighten

"Rainbow!" I say out loud, any time I spot a rainbow, regardless of who I'm with (or if I'm on my own). I am still flabbergasted by rainbows. How? Why? Multiple colours in the sky because of a combination of sunshine and water molecules? Magical!

And if the rainbow happens to brighten instead of fade, if the arc lengthens and stretches across the sky, well! Doesn't that feel about as close to a miracle as you are likely to experience in everyday life?

Similar glimmers:
+ *The sun peeking through the clouds after rain.*
+ *Cloud gazing.*

Hearing an owl hoot

There is so much going on in the natural world that people have no idea about. So many mysterious creatures living their lives, oblivious to humans, under cover of darkness, or far away from light and noise, deep underwater or deep in the bush. An owl hooting in the pitch black of night is a good reminder that there's more to the world than meets the eye.

Similar glimmers:
+ *Spotting dolphins as you look out at the ocean.*
+ *Discovering an intricate bird's nest.*

Ordinary sunrises and sunsets

I would like to say a word in praise of ordinary sunrises and sunsets. Isn't it remarkable that the sun rises and sets every single day? And there is beauty in each of these. Maybe not gasp-worthy beauty, but beauty nonetheless. Anything that connects you to awe – whether it's Awe with a capital A, or just a whispered moment of it – is good for your mental health, and your daily life.

Similar glimmers:
+ *Being inside, watching a storm.*
+ *Slow, spectacular sunsets. You take a photo, thinking this is as good as it gets. A few minutes later, it's even better, so you take another one, and so on.*

Freshly mown grass

Walking past a freshly mown lawn and inhaling deeply is probably one of the quickest and cheapest ways to appreciate being alive. It's so green. So fresh! So often effortless for you: a chance encounter with lawn mowing day for somebody else.

Similar glimmers:
+ *Inhaling deeply as you enter a bakery.*
+ *Breathing in great lungfuls of pine-scented air in a wood or forest.*

A butterfly dancing in the air

There's the street, the pavement, the grass, the trees, all the same as they were yesterday. And then, suddenly! A butterfly, flitting about. Dancing along to some unheard tune. Brightly coloured, or brown, or black and white, it makes no difference: there is something inherently joyful about watching a butterfly.

Similar glimmers:
+ *The hum of bees buzzing in a bush.*
+ *A dragonfly skimming across the water.*

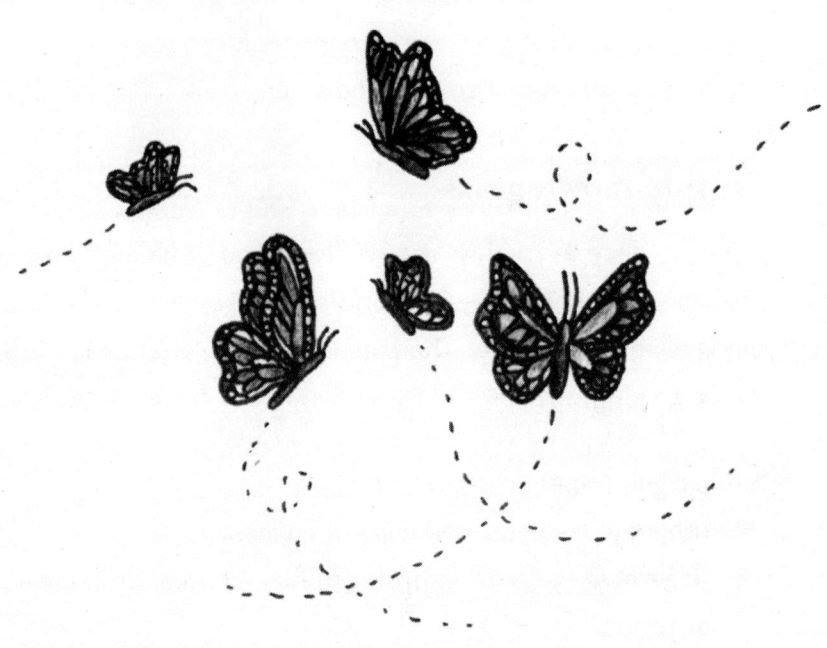

Tame nature

When I talk about glimmers in nature, it's not all mountains and rivers and wild rocky outcrops. There is as much joy to be found in a kitchen pot plant, or a window box with a few herbs. City birds are birds nonetheless, and insects thrive in all kinds of settings. Sometimes you need to take the magnifying glass a little closer to connect with the wonder of nature in the middle of city life, but it's there all the same.

Similar glimmers:
+ *Morning light slanting in and making house plants glow.*
+ *The first flower on a plant you're growing.*

Watching birds fly

Imagine a world without birds! No birdsong, no watching birds fly through the skies, no twittering and chirping ... We have a bottlebrush tree outside our bedroom window, and one of my favourite ways to start the day is to watch the hummingbirds flit about the tree, gathering nectar. It's endlessly entertaining and soothing.

Similar glimmers:
+ *Watching a hawk circle high up in the sky.*
+ *Watching birds try to balance on a wire in the wind.*

Awe walks

An awe walk doesn't have to be a big production. It can simply be going for a walk with your senses tuned for anything that might spark a little awe. Not mouth-hanging-open wonder, simply a moment of, "Wow." A small, quiet amazement.

Similar glimmers:
+ *Hiking a new nature trail.*
+ *Having a ladybird or ladybug (both names are sheer delight!) land on you.*

The nature trail nod

I have gone on nature walks all around the world, and I can tell you that one thing remains the same, no matter what country you're in: there is an acknowledgement, a greeting between walkers or hikers on these trails that seems to span all cultures.

Some of the greeters are more enthusiastic, of course (here's looking at you, America!), but the consistent habit of a nod or smile as you pass each other makes it feel like one big nature rambling club. And that is very sweet.

Similar glimmers:
+ *Finding a woodland scene that looks like a fairy dwelling.*
+ *Mist amid trees.*

Sipping on a cuppa while looking at the sky

Most mornings, let's be frank, do not begin with an abundance of calm. But on those special mornings when you can pause to sip your tea or coffee, while watching streaks of light and colour paint across the sky like watercolours from an unseen hand, it is a beautiful way to start the day.

Similar glimmers:
+ *Dappled sunshine.*
+ *Gazing out at the ocean.*

Feeding crumbs to a bird

You spot a bird, hopping around, pretending not to look at your sandwich, biscuit, cracker or whatever you're eating. You crumble up a morsel and toss it into the space between you. A look, a few hops, a shy peck and whoosh, the bird has taken its prize. Only to return a moment later, looking for more.

It's a strange and lovely dance between human and animal, and it's taking place in cities and towns and villages all over the world, every day.

Similar glimmers:
+ *The wonder of gladioli and larkspur opening, slowly unfurling and getting more exquisite every day.*
+ *Sitting in the leafy shade sipping tea.*

An extraordinary view

Whenever I visit somebody who lives in a home with an extraordinary view, I always ask if they get used to it. They often say yes. Repetition tends to dull the senses, regardless of splendour.

But to chance upon an extraordinary view for the first time is a striking thing. It's a moment of pause in the frenzy of life, a discrete slice of time – no matter how thin – to ground yourself in the present moment. Look at that! Wow.

Similar glimmers:

✦ *Dawn. The darkness shifts to a dull grey, which lightens until – look! Is that some colour? The colours brighten and deepen until the sun starts rising and suddenly, it's day.*

✦ *Dusk. The brightness of full daylight fades so slowly sometimes that it's hard to tell exactly when it transitions into dusk, except that the colours are softer and everything looks more peaceful. And then, within a few moments, darkness.*

Watching a leaf fall gently from a tree

It happens every day, but in the rush of everyday life, you often don't see leaves falling. Which is what makes the moment of noticing so special. A leaf chooses this one moment to detach and float gently down to the ground in a pirouette or a dive, a hover or a sail. It's a moment of presence.

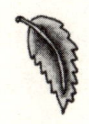

Similar glimmers:
+ *The way trees reflect in still water.*
+ *Standing in the middle of a ring of trees.*

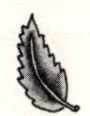

Planting a tree

You've probably heard the Chinese proverb: "The best time to plant a tree was 20 years ago. The second best time is now." Planting a tree feels like one of the kindest things you can do: for yourself, for the future and for the environment.

Similar glimmers:
+ *The satisfying heft of a spade when you dig it into soil to plant something.*
+ *Sinking your hands into the earth.*

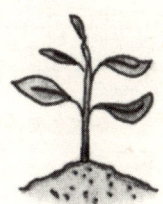

Limitless horizons

I am a firm believer in the power of limitless horizons to calm the mind and boost mental and emotional wellbeing. The ocean is the ultimate limitless horizon, but lakes, deserts, fields and mountains all count too. Whatever makes you feel expansive and like the world is full of possibility. Whatever lets your eyes rest and your mind exhale.

Similar glimmers:
+ *Sunshine on a wave that's just receding and leaving glistening wet sand behind it.*
+ *Shadow play from a branch of leaves dancing in the wind.*

Spotting a wild creature on a nature walk

This will vary dramatically depending where in the world you are. You could be talking monkeys, squirrels, owls, birds of prey or deer. Regardless of type, it is thrilling to spot a wild creature, any wild creature, while you're out on a nature walk. Some greater connection to Nature with a capital N that calls to you, and you find it answers back.

Similar glimmers:
+ *Getting lost on a trail, and then finding your way back again.*
+ *Seeing a whale surface and spout air.*

The top of the mountain

You're out of breath. Your calves are screaming. Your feet feel like you've been walking for days. But you've done it! As you crest the mountain and look out over the view, it all feels worth it. You're on top of the world!

Similar glimmers:
+ *The light hitting the mountains, just so.*
+ *Snorkelling or scuba diving – a whole world beneath the waves.*

Swimming in a lake

Swimming in a lake feels very primal. That fresh, earthy water smell. The squelch of mud as you wade in (not a favourite for many, I know) and then the push off into the middle of the lake, where you can float on your back and gaze upward, or dive underwater into the bluey green.

For those who think this sounds one step above "no thanks", maybe a boat trip might work for you, instead?

Similar glimmers:
+ *Walking into a warm ocean that's so clear you can see your toes.*
+ *Swimming or boating in a river that's burbling happily, with no strong currents to be seen.*

A day of rain after a long dry spell

If you've ever lived through a drought, you will know the sweet, profound relief when rain suddenly starts falling. The ground is so thirsty you can almost hear it sucking up the water.

But it's the same with any extended weather pattern, isn't it? If it's been cloudy or rainy for weeks, the chance of the sun coming out and revealing a blue sky is wonderful. Sometimes you need to live through the bad weather to truly understand the joy of a lovely day.

Similar glimmers:
+ *A day of sunshine after a day of non-stop rain.*
+ *The sound of gentle morning rain.*

Planting seedlings

Is there anything as hopeful as planting seedlings? It feels like planting hope. Taking the delicate little seedlings out of their container and nesting them in a pot or plot, patting the soil down around them, giving them a little drink of water. It's an investment in the future – no matter how small that investment might seem.

Similar glimmers:
+ *Planting cuttings from a friend's garden.*
+ *Repotting house plants.*

Watching a river in full flow

Watching a river in full flow is entrancing. The power of it, the force ... particularly if you're standing on a bridge, and can drop little sticks in to watch them get whisked away.

Similar glimmers:
+ *A budding flower on a plant you thought was dead.*
+ *Drinking water from a waterfall (very oxygenated!).*

Petrichor: the scent of rain on hot earth

Sometimes a word just hits the spot. Petrichor is one of those: the earthy green smell when rain falls on hot earth.

Similar glimmers:
+ *A swim in a clear mountain pool.*
+ *Being in nature, with no other humans around.*

Golden hour

The day has come to an end. It's the golden hour: the hour when photos look their best and capture people with an inner glow. The hour when you get to pause, exhale and regroup.

Similar glimmers:
+ *Birdsong at dusk.*
+ *Cicadas singing on a summer night.*

Poking around in a rock pool

A rock pool is a microcosm of the ocean. It is remarkable that you can look in one and get to see all the different colours, creatures, rocks and shells up close. If you're looking for a micro-dose of awe, look no further than a rock pool.

Similar glimmers:
+ *A tree laden with blossoms.*
+ *A fresh mountain breeze that carries the scent of high peaks and wildness.*

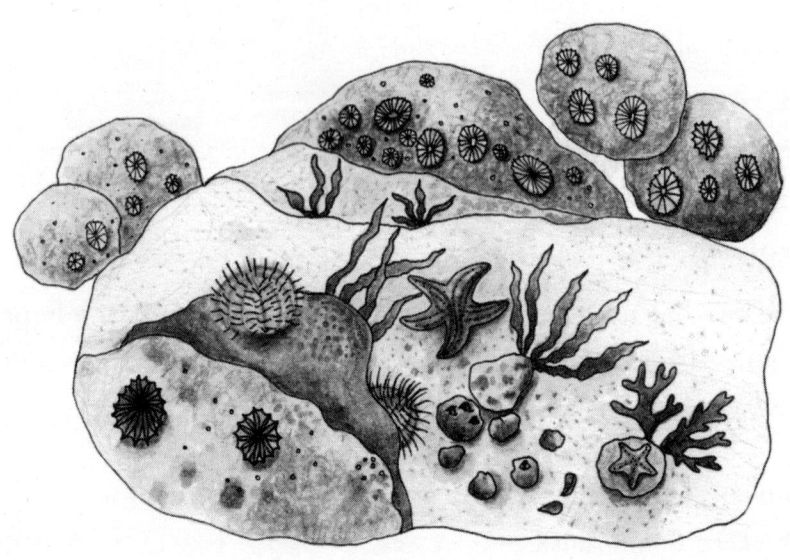

Surprised by a full moon

You glance out the window and – there! Like a scene from a gothic horror novel, the giant moon is rising. It does this every month, of course, but if you're like me, you're often glued to your phone or TV or so deep in conversation that you don't even notice. When you do take the time to watch the moon rise, it is every bit as beautiful and majestic as you remembered. And it connects you (and me) somehow, to something bigger, something mystical and primal and real.

Similar glimmers:
+ *Stargazing. Preferably wrapped up in a blanket, lying next to someone you love, but really any time spent staring at the night sky is time well-spent.*
+ *Spotting a shooting star.*

New leaves on a previously sad tree

You think the tree is a goner. And then, out of nowhere, something that looks like a bud ... and that bud unfurls into a leaf, and suddenly there is hope and life and renewal and wellbeing when all of that was lost.

Similar glimmers:
+ *Flowering plant boxes on a city street.*
+ *Chancing on a waterfall, however small.*

Walking on the beach

The lapping waves on the shore, the feel of soft beach sand or stones beneath your feet, the limitless horizon – wonderful.

If you're more of a mountain person who loves mountain biking, you do you. A desert person who loves yoga? Sounds awesome. Anything that combines some kind of movement with some kind of natural beauty is what you're looking for here. A big ol' slice of joy.

Similar glimmers:
+ *Space to run as far as you want.*
+ *Finding natural treasures, like a shell or some sea glass, on the beach.*

The smell of a botanical garden

No matter where in the world the botanical garden is, some things will be consistent. It will be green green green. It will be filled with many attractive plants and trees, and some truly unusual and eye-catching plants and trees. And it will smell … familiar. Like earth and loam and growing and hope.

Similar glimmers:
+ *A rainbow caught in a spray of water.*
+ *The wonder of wisteria, exploding like flowery fireworks.*

Apricity: the warmth of the sun on a cold day

It hardly feels related to the summer sun because its warmth is so mild in comparison, but there is something truly, bodily comforting about rays of autumn and winter sun soaking into your chilled bones. The fact that there's such a pretty word for it is just a bonus!

Similar glimmers:
+ *Basking in sunshine. Basking, friends! Basking.*
+ *Bad weather lifting long enough to enjoy the outdoors (albeit briefly).*

Extraordinary trees

There are some truly crazy trees in this world. The sausage tree grows a poisonous fruit that looks exactly like a sausage. The dragon's blood tree has sap as red as blood. The bottle tree looks like somebody made a tree out of a bottle, without changing its shape at all. And the rainbow eucalyptus sheds bark in red, blue, pink, orange, yellow and green.

Similar glimmers:
+ *Wild flowers that erupt in abundance.*
+ *The unassuming majesty of old trees.*

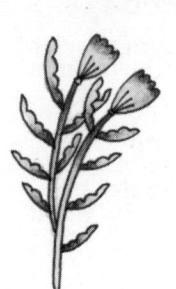

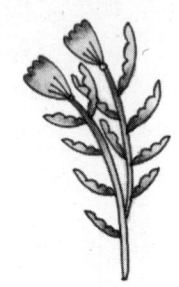

ONE GOOD THING
A DAY

A really useful practice to get into is "one good thing a day". The idea is to find one good thing that happens every day, and share it at the dinner table, or write it down if you live alone. I do this with my husband and kids every day, and it is reliably one of my daily glimmers: even if we've all had kind of an average day, the storytelling brings us together.

And there's always something that you can find as your good thing. Some days this will be easy: something fun happened, or you achieved something, or someone brought surprise birthday cake to work or school. Other days, it's a challenge.

The blah days are when this practice is most important. Because even on the most blah day, there is a slice or two of joy. Remember, you're just looking for three-second moments: the bar is extremely low.

"I was cold and I put a warm top on." That's a slice of joy.

"I got home, took my shoes off and sat on the couch." That's one good thing.

There's an accountability factor here too. Knowing that you have to report on one good thing at dinner tunes your senses toward noticing glimmers. It makes you more alert and aware of tiny pleasing moments. And that, inevitably, improves your day. (The bonus is that it also reveals a lot about the people you're having dinner with.)

Try it for a week, and see how you feel ...

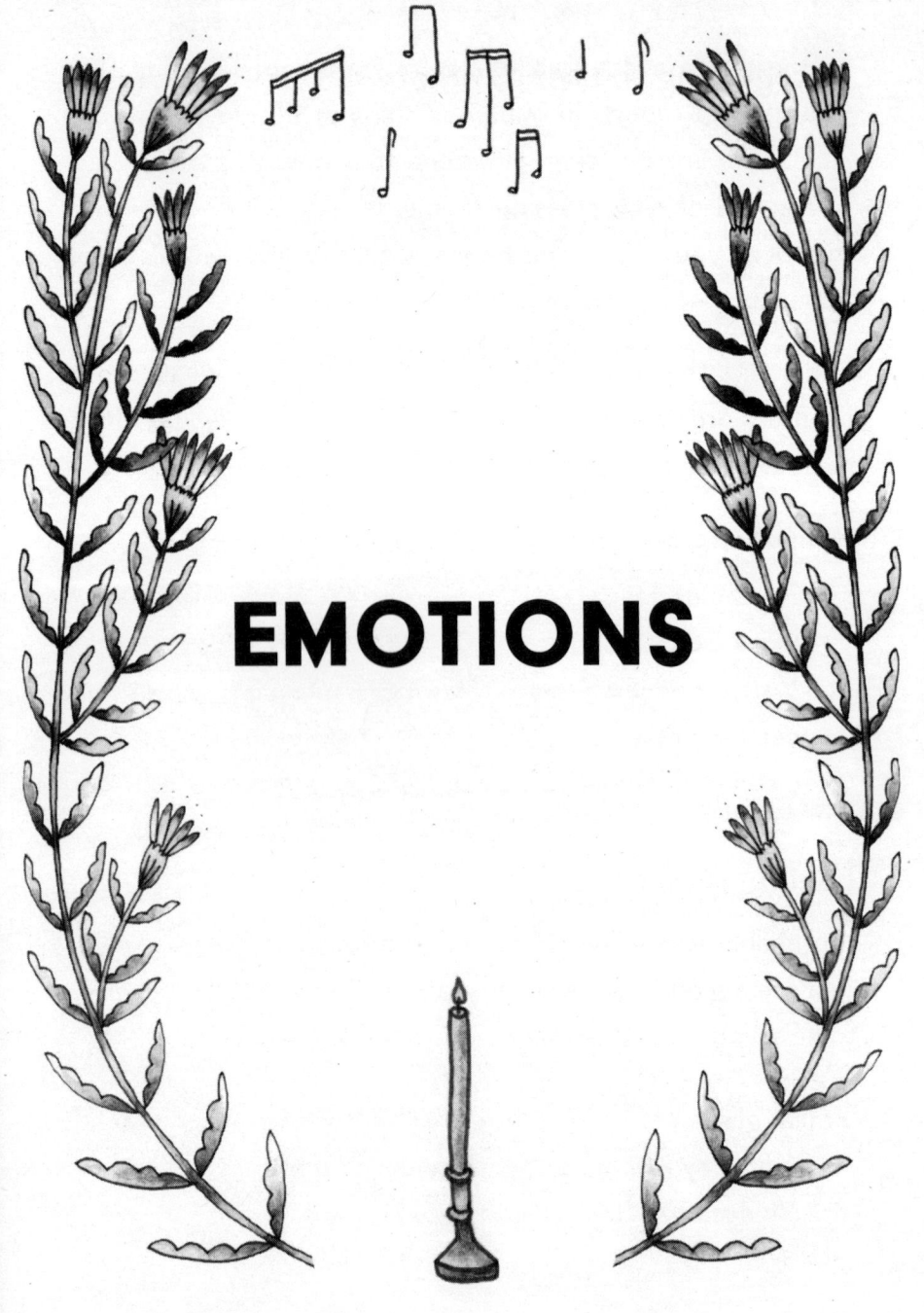

EMOTIONS

Recognizing the beautiful ordinary

The beautiful ordinary is recognizing how lovely this, right here, is. Sure, it's nothing special, but isn't it so nice that you can be reading these words in the relative comfort of wherever you are right now? At first, it might seem like an uncomfortable habit to get into, making a hero out of a moment that is not very special. But with time, all those beautiful ordinary moments add up and it becomes clear that each of those tiny glimmers was a hero, in its own right.

Similar glimmers:
✦ *Feeling useful. Get stuck into something (anything!) and make a difference, no matter how small.*
✦ *Visible kindness – a smile, a note, a hug, a gift, a task quietly crossed off your list without you having to ask, a cup of tea just the way you like it.*

Feeling relaxed

It probably says something about the speed of life these days that feeling relaxed is a novelty, but it is! A wonderful novelty, to be savoured and remarked upon and treasured.

Similar glimmers:
✦ *A holiday with long days of no obligations.*
✦ *No need to get out of bed until you want to.*

Cheerful anticipation (of anything)

"I can't wait for …!" You think, and a little internal shiver of anticipation runs through you. It might be a special dinner, a weekend away, a fun date with friends, a live show … It's so lovely to have something to look forward to, big or small. More of these moments, please.

Similar glimmers:
+ *Planning a birthday cake with a child.*
+ *Freshly popped popcorn, perfectly seasoned, and a movie you know you'll love.*

Feeling calm in a usually stressful situation

There is deep satisfaction when you realize that you are handling a situation well. Particularly if you are managing to stay calm in a stressful situation: remembering to breathe, recognizing that there are many things beyond your control, and pausing before you react. All the good stuff that you know but somehow fail to integrate, usually.

Similar glimmers:
+ *Centring yourself.*
+ *Doing a meditation, where you think of someone you love and then radiate that love out to your family, friends, colleagues, strangers, town, country and the world.*

A safe space to unpack thoughts and feelings

You're feeling ... something. Something big and complex and unwieldy. It would be so helpful to lay it all out, in front of a (gentle) witness and see if the pieces make sense in some way. And then you are given that space, from a therapist, a friend, a colleague, a partner. What a relief.

Similar glimmers:
+ *(Happily) admitting you were wrong.*
+ *Learning more about a topic you really care about.*

Expert reassurance on a life decision

You've decided to Do It (whatever It is) and you're 90 per cent sure it's the right decision, but not 100 per cent certain because who can ever be totally certain in this life, really? You explain your reasoning to someone you respect, who you believe has a thorough understanding of the situation, and they assure you that you have, indeed, made the right decision. Hooray!

Similar glimmers:
+ *An incisive question that gets to the heart of what you're trying to figure out.*
+ *Making a decision quickly and easily because the answer seems so clear.*

JOMO (the Joy Of Missing Out)

Your friends are out doing something fun, but you listened to your body and stayed home instead. You're curled up in pyjamas, watching a movie and you couldn't be happier. This, friends, is JOMO.

Similar glimmers:

+ *Any kind of abundance: good things to eat, excellent shows to watch or lovely people to see. That overflowing feeling of good fortune.*
+ *Enthusiasm, in all its forms. Feeling fired up to do something, and expressing it.*

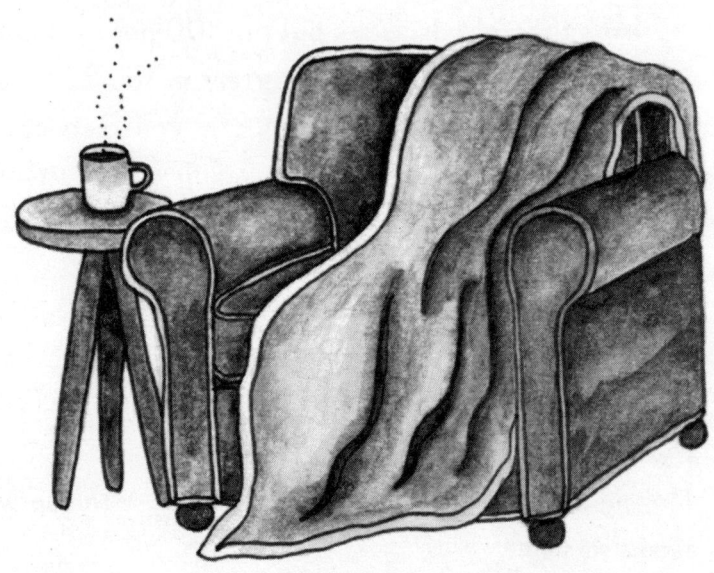

Walking down a (short) memory lane

Walking down memory lane can be bittersweet, or deliciously sweet or totally bitter. But if you time it right, a short memory lane meander will give you just the hit you need: a few poignant memories, a reminder of how far you've come, and an appreciation both for the past and for the fact that it has passed.

Similar glimmers:

+ *Returning to a once-familiar spot to find how much you've changed.*
+ *Commemorating a personally life-changing anniversary.*

The excitement of planning a holiday

Oh, the potential wonders that await you when you plan a holiday! Especially in the initial phase, when it's not even about a real holiday, just the various lives you'd like to live for a few days. Where might you go? What might you do? The options are endless ...

Similar glimmers:

+ *Gathering wood for a bonfire: the anticipation of the blaze when it's dark enough to light all that wood.*
+ *The first morning of a holiday, when potential fun stretches ahead of you.*

Stepping outside your emotional comfort zone

Your emotional comfort zone is your safe space: where your feelings are predictable and familiar, even if they're not always positive. Your comfort zone is there for a reason – to let you function as a (mostly) normal adult. But sometimes it can grow a little stifling and start resembling more of a rut. That's when it's time to climb, briefly, into something new. Even if it makes you a little uncertain or anxious; even if it feels like something you haven't done before and you're not entirely sure you *can* do. You don't have to stay out there for long: just long enough to show yourself how malleable you truly are.

Similar glimmers:
+ *Stepping back into your comfort zone.*
+ *Recognizing that you are not the person you used to be.*

Some time at home alone

There is such peace in being able to do exactly what you want in your own home. Nobody to answer to, or explain your actions. No need to think about if you're being productive or using your time well. Simply space to be yourself.

Similar glimmers:
+ *Looking out at a still, calm view.*
+ *A long, slow journey by yourself.*

Lowering your bar for gratitude

I love the idea of a low bar for gratitude. The more easily pleased you are, the more joyful your life will be. The first hot shower when your plumbing is fixed? Blissful.

Similar glimmers:
+ *The relief of the-day-after-stomach-bug.*
+ *Surprised by something in everyday life.*

Being able to laugh at yourself

Humans are such silly creatures sometimes. You and I will inevitably do something daft this week – say something ridiculous, make a faux pas of some description – and almost as inevitably try to cover it up. But what if you didn't? What if you owned the ridiculous and laughed at yourself in a carefree way? When you can truly laugh at yourself – truly see the funny in whoever is making fun, and recognize that (unless they are bad people) they aren't trying to be unkind – that is such a freeing discovery. It also means more laughter in your life, which is always a good thing.

Similar glimmers:
+ *Cackling with laughter.*
+ *Serendipity: the specific delight of some good luck crossing your path at precisely the right time.*

A fresh new beginning

Today is the first day of the rest of your life. You know this. I know this. You will never be this young again, or have so much life ahead to live. Your life begins anew today. What are you going to do with it?

Similar glimmers:
+ *"They're here!"*
+ *The promise of new library books, magazines or episodes of your favourite TV show – whatever you look forward to diving into.*

Alignment

Everything seems to be going your way. You're well-rested. You're healthy. Work is going well. Family life is going well. Nobody is ill. There's nothing majorly disruptive on the horizon. Just for now, just for today, all is in alignment. And glory be, it is remarkable!

Similar glimmers:
+ *Recognition of a life well-lived, of someone's pleasant behaviour or of a good deed. Such a lovely feeling.*
+ *Peace. Rare, fleeting and precious.*

Booking tickets for something fun

It could be a comedian, a music show, a movie you've been wanting to watch or a trip to the theatre. Regardless, you're looking forward to it, and it's on the horizon. How fun to wait in cheerful anticipation!

Similar glimmers:
+ *Paying for a getaway (holiday confirmed, whoop whoop!).*
+ *Looking forward to a day out, somewhere local and low-key.*

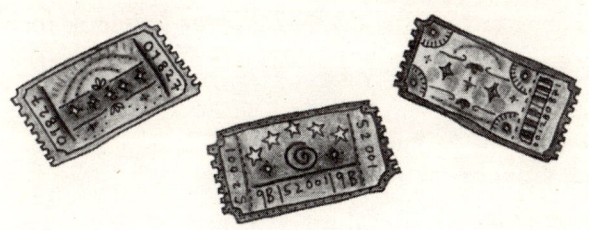

Making an impact

Humans are meaning-seeking creatures. One of the most direct avenues to meaning is feeling that your presence, your efforts and your actions are having an effect and changing something for someone. That's a great big slice of joy.

Similar glimmers:
+ *Coming up with a solution that solves a problem.*
+ *Being challenged in just the right way, so you feel mentally sharpened or creatively inspired.*

Completing the stress response cycle

I was first introduced to the stress response cycle by Emily and Amelia Nagoski in their book *Burnout*.[25] Essentially, any time you are stressed, there is a stressor and a stress response. Once the stressor lifts (you hand in the assignment, get out of traffic, finish the argument ...), the stress response needs to be completed in order to return the body to calm. It's a physical reaction and it needs a physical resolution. You can complete the stress response cycle in seven ways:

1. Movement and exercise
2. A 20-second hug
3. Deep, slow breathing
4. Casual, friendly social interaction
5. Laughing
6. Crying
7. Creative expression of any kind

You'll probably have favourite ways to get the stress out of your body. I like dancing or going for a fast walk. Once you learn how to complete the cycle, it's remarkable the difference it can make. Like emptying a bucket before it overflows.

Similar glimmers:
+ *Feeling at home, whatever that feeling means to you.*
+ *Being honest about how you feel, even if that's hard.*

The relief when a health scare is just a scare

My dad has had more than his fair share of health scares. You know the ones when two paths open up in front of you, and one is so awful and the other one is just fine. As a result, I am now acutely aware of the grace that follows a health scare that doesn't turn into anything more. It feels like a gift from the heavens, and can realign you to the blessing of ordinary good health.

You know how it goes: you're asked to do further tests, and then you wait for the results and imagine your two possible futures. And then! Glory be, it was just a scare. Thank heavens.

Similar glimmers:
+ *Skating over the top of a cold – when you think you're getting sick, and then a good night's rest fixes it.*
+ *"Well, that went surprisingly well!"*

That moment when the lights dim in a cinema

You've watched the trailers and the ads, eaten most of your snacks and then the lights dim ... The film's starting!

Similar glimmers:
+ *The moment the curtain lifts in a theatre.*
+ *That feeling of excitement when you're hiding in a game of hide-and-seek and nobody has found you yet.*

Respair: a return to hope

Isn't that a lovely word: respair? And a similarly lovely feeling: when it seems possible to dare hope again. Perhaps things won't be as desperate as you feared; perhaps they might even work themselves out.

Similar glimmers:
+ *Seeing a light at the end of the tunnel. At last!*
+ *Feeling giddy.*

Golden-hued memories

It is remarkable that you can differentiate between memories, if you think about it. You've been gathering them since you were a child. Your memory bank must surely be overloaded. And yet, in among all those memories there are the golden-hued ones: moments that stand out and make you smile, no matter how old they are.

Even if the memory is tinged with sadness because of what came afterward, that doesn't take the golden edge off it. Somehow it makes it shine brighter.

Similar glimmers:
+ *Specific photos that spark cherished childhood memories.*
+ *Eating your favourite treat from when you were a kid, and still liking the taste.*

Coming home after a busy outing

You've been out and about: seeing people, doing things, living life. And then you come home, and it's quiet and peaceful. You have some time to recalibrate, a pause to exhale.

Similar glimmers:
+ *Making peace (sometimes alongside the person you're making peace with, sometimes on your own).*
+ *Contentment. The most underrated of all the happiness forms and yet, I think, perhaps the most valuable.*

A song that feels made for you

In this moment, right now. The music plays, and your reaction is a whole body "Yes".

Similar glimmers:
+ *Possibilities – like twinkling stars, they glitter just ahead. Which one will come to fruition? It's hard to know, but the fact that they are there is thrilling in its own way. You get to experience all the wonder of unrealized potential without any of the hard work (yet).*
+ *Clarity. Things have been murky and confusing, and then – either by doing some specific work or letting some time pass – clarity emerges. The path forward is clear.*

Laughing unexpectedly

So unexpectedly you spit out whatever is in your mouth, and then proceed to choke a little, gasping for breath as you carry on laughing, trying not to pee your pants.

Similar glimmers:
+ *Feeling like a kid.*
+ *Those rare moments when you're not thinking about the past or the future but just perfectly, presently, here.*

Candlelit yoga

Candlelit anything is great. Even better if it's soothing, relaxing and an opportunity for you to focus on your breath and your body. Just for a while, you don't have to think of anything beyond that.

Similar glimmers:
+ *Savasana at the end of a yoga class. Everyone lying down, relaxing.*
+ *Bedtime. The day is done. You've done your best (or not so much) and there's nothing more to do but tuck yourself in and rest.*

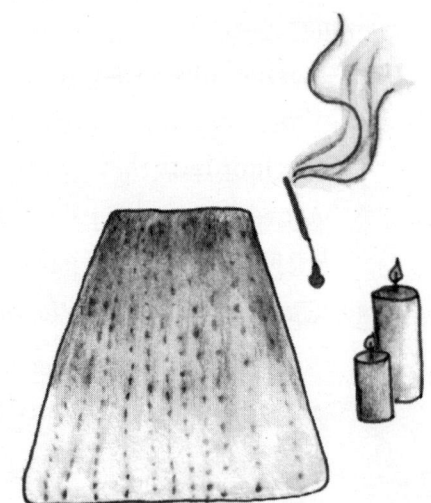

A free afternoon

"What are you up to this afternoon?"
"Nothing much ..."

Ah ... the beauty of nothing much! Time to do exactly as you please! Think of the possibilities, or the deep peace of doing nothing at all.

Similar glimmers:
+ *A relaxed morning: no alarm, no plans.*
+ *Lazy Sunday lunch with friends: nothing but time unspooling ahead of you.*

Eyes full of love

Considering how often humans look at each other, it's somewhat surprising how unusual this is, and yet it's rare enough to notice when someone looks at you and there's pure love pouring out of their eyes. What a special feeling.

Similar glimmers:
+ *A loved one asking how you are – and really wanting to know the answer.*
+ *Looking at someone you love and feeling your heart swell.*

Forgiveness

Forgiveness can be so hard. Especially if you're on a high horse of judgement and the other person truly deserves not to be forgiven for their dastardly behaviour. Luckily, time passes. You work through your feelings and hopefully, one day, walk your way into forgiveness.

Similar glimmers:

+ *Acceptance. "Everything in time and on time and for the greater good of all," is one of my favourite mantras. And some days, magically, I believe it.*
+ *Calm. Things are happening: stressful things, upsetting things, noisy things. You are doing your best to manage them but more importantly, somehow, you are remaining calm. Like the still centre of a hurricane, calm prevails.*

Collective effervescence

I love everything about collective effervescence ... people fizzing gently together, that energy and harmony when you're in a crowd and you're all feeling the same thing at the same time.

Similar glimmers:

+ *Being part of a standing ovation.*
+ *Watching a band you love perform live – that soaring feeling in your chest.*

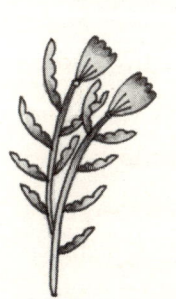

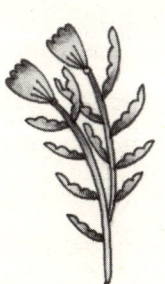

SLICES OF JOY,
NO MATTER WHAT

Noticing glimmers and crafting slices of joy doesn't presuppose that everything in your life is peachy. Remember, glimmers are micro-moments of nervous system regulation: if everything was easy, fun and happy all the time, your nervous system wouldn't need regulating. Ross Gay said it succinctly: "Joy has nothing to do with ease. Joy has everything to do with the fact that we're all going to die."[26]

If it was one rainbow cupcake after another, one delightful, seamless life experience followed by a nap and then another delight, what would any of it mean? The beauty comes from the fact that you are given this moment, now, and then it is gone, forever.

Joy is most powerful within a backdrop of arduous things, in fact, because life is filled with arduous things – people getting sick, and dying, relationships ending and work drying up, friendships faltering and finances running out. Slices of joy, in spite of. Slices of joy, no matter what.

✦ The joy of the Stoics

The Stoics wrote about joy a lot. They've got a bad reputation, I know, and I think that's largely because being a Stoic has been equated with having a stiff upper lip, and not expressing many emotions. But actually, Seneca – the first of the three great Stoic philosophers (Seneca, Epictetus and Marcus Aurelius), born way back in 4 BCE – said that someone who practises Stoicism "desires no joys greater than his inner joys", and if that isn't a fancy way of saying enjoy what you have right in front of you, I don't know what is!

Much of the Stoic way of life is about quelling desires. They want to reduce the constant wanting of things you don't have, and the desire to control everything. Minimizing that feeling of desperate wanting leads to a far more peaceful life, where joy is more likely to be found.

In William B. Irvine's wonderful book on Stoicism in modern life, *A Guide to the Good Life*, he speaks about how practising Stoicism can make you "susceptible to little outbursts of joy"[27], carried on a wave of gratitude and a recognition of the good fortune of being who you are, living your life right now.

Let me give you an example of Stoicism in action. I got stuck in a terrible traffic jam (a 30-minute delay, desperately needed to pee, really hungry for lunch). But instead of ranting and raging, as I usually do in traffic, I rolled my window down. Appreciated the trees and mountains that

I usually can't see because I'm zooming past. Listened to a truly outstanding podcast – really listened, because I wasn't moving. When I eventually got home, I felt calm. After I peed, I felt borderline euphoric (if you know, you know). And when I ate lunch, at last, I felt truly grateful for it.

You know the feeling: you're stuck in a situation and your blood starts boiling. But if you can truly accept what is in and out of your control, that's where the glimmers lie. The Stoics wrote about three kinds of situation:

1. Those you have no control over (such as traffic)
2. Those you have limited control over (trying your best)
3. Those you have complete control over (your goals and values)

So often, you spend large chunks of your time getting upset about things over which you have no control. (So do I.) Stoicism suggests that if you value tranquillity, this is a futile pursuit. I love this because it's such a clear-eyed view of the world. It takes away the desire for things to be different, and focuses the attention on how things actually are.

✦ Right here, right now

The goal is finding delight in what is right here, right now, and managing your wants to below your needs. What does that mean? Only wanting what you already have. In fact, wanting less than you already have, thereby feeling delighted and lucky by the abundance in your life. That's where contentment lies.

Writer Sara Ahmed said, "Where we find happiness teaches us what we value rather than simply what is of value," and I think that sums it up so perfectly.[28] The recipe for slices of joy will be different for each person. What lifts my heart might not have any impact on yours – and that's totally fine. What matters is that you're on the lookout, and that you're aware you'll find it inside. There's no striving, here. No external validation. What a blessed relief.

✦ Delicious attention

Maybe, in fact, this practice is less about reaching for joy and more about allowing it in. Meditation teacher Shivani Ranchod offers a reminder that, "Inviting joy into our lives requires paying closer attention: slowing down to make noticing possible. And practising directing our attention towards things that are beautiful, things that are astonishing, things that are surprising, things that are delicious."

It really is about where you direct your attention: what you choose to pay attention to (and where it is being stolen from you with your full permission – here's looking at you, social media!). Where are you spending your delicious attention? Are you doing it purposefully?

✦ A rigorous discipline of joy

How do we ensure we find this joy, though? Even in very privileged spaces (I count myself as the lucky resident of one of these), joy can be elusive and difficult to hold on to. It's so easy to get sucked into the daily humdrum of stresses, deadlines and duties. And while everyday stress may seem like a "nice problem" to have (in comparison to some of the stressors that others are living through), that doesn't stop it from being real, and true for many people. There's no competition for who is having the hardest time, is there? No ranking where you can decide if your pain is worthy. If you are struggling, you're struggling: regardless of whether or not you "should" be.

The writer and mystic Andrew Harvey suggests "a rigorous discipline of joy". That might sound a little hard and unyielding, but the concept is sound. In the same way that you have to exercise to build muscles so that you can do things you couldn't do before, you have to practise (there's that word again!) building the joy muscle. You don't merely wake up and feel joyful, most of the time. Maybe if it's your birthday or you're on holiday, or A Good Thing just happened. But many days there's a scrolling To Do List, something serious to grapple with, a concern or two calling for your attention. Ensuring joy is on that list, even if only for a few moments, is essential.

✦ Let's start at the end

Contemplating death, can (paradoxically) lead to a quiet sense of joy. The Stoics practise *Memento Mori*, Latin for "remember you must die", as a meditation on the inevitability of death. While that may sound really depressing, it is actually a life-affirming exercise.

The idea is that every day, for two or three minutes, you choose something you love (your health, your partner, your child, your job ...) and contemplate what your life would be like if you were to lose it. You don't "plug in" to the feeling: the idea isn't to emotionally connect and get upset, but rather to think through how your life would be different. When you emerge from the meditation, you have a renewed appreciation for whatever it was you contemplated losing. Suddenly your partner is less irritating, your job less boring and your child less demanding.

You're simply, presently, aware of your good fortune. Noticing the glimmers.

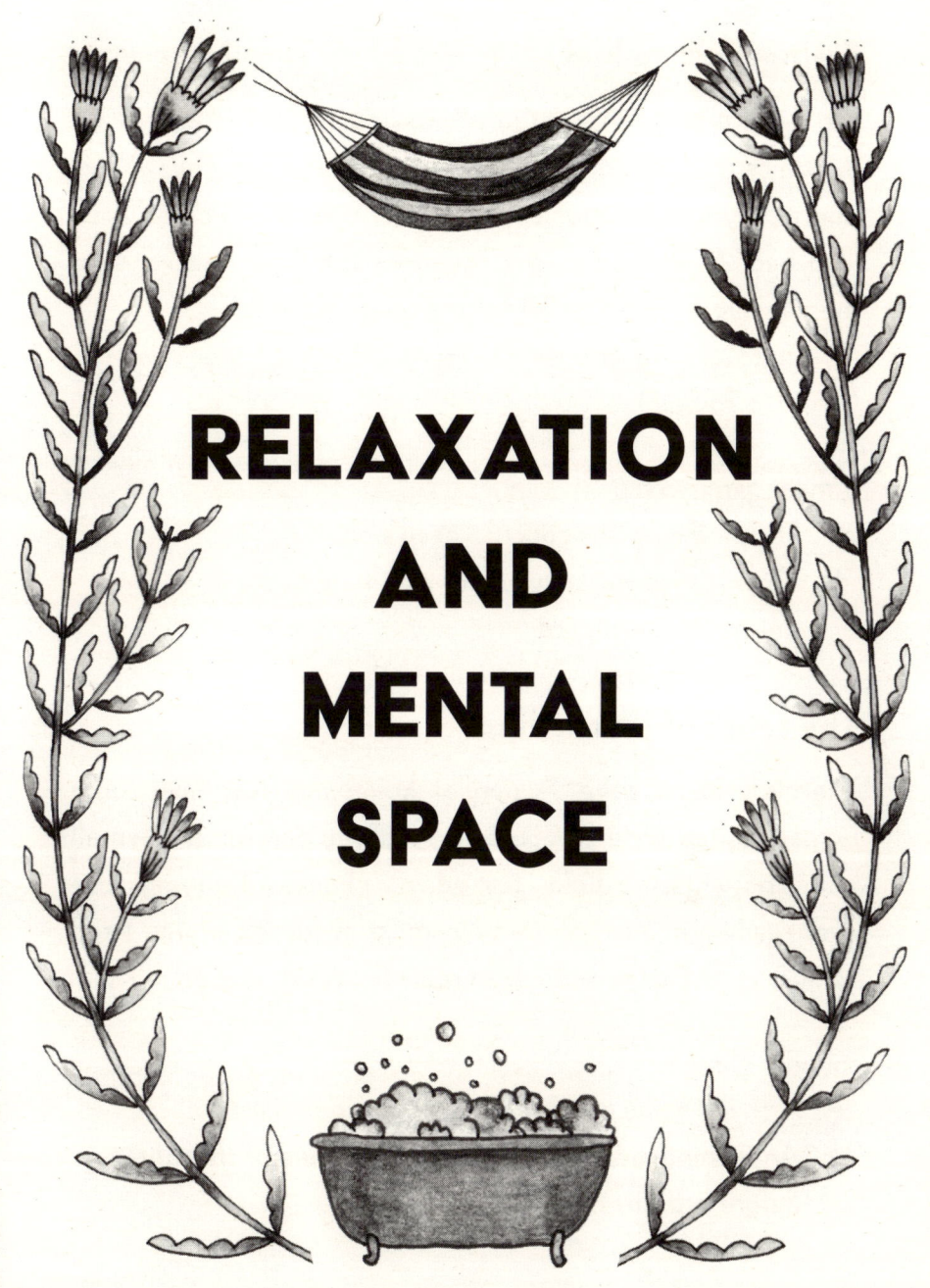

RELAXATION AND MENTAL SPACE

Going back to bed

It's been a busy week. You've worked so hard. You have a bunch of things to do today, but just for an extra cheeky five minutes, you take your cup of tea or coffee and climb back into bed. Maybe pick up a book, or stare out the window, message your friend or listen to a song you love.

Whatever you choose to do, this five minutes is a PTS (Present To Self).

Similar glimmers:
+ *Flopping onto the couch ... deep sigh.*
+ *An unrushed weekday lunch, with time to chew slowly, uninterrupted.*

The relief of journalling

There's a blank page. A pen or keyboard. You have some uninterrupted time to yourself. And you can write down all your thoughts, no-holds-barred, no chance of anyone else ever reading it. You can be your most awful self, if you need to, just on the page and not in real life. What a relief!

Similar glimmers:
+ *Arriving home after getting soaked in a rainstorm.*
+ *An evening meditation to clear your mind of thoughts before bedtime.*

Time off

Whether it's a holiday, a long weekend, or simply an afternoon to yourself, time off does exactly what it says on the box: gives you a break from the daily grind. Could you give yourself 20 minutes of time off today?

Similar glimmers:
+ *A long walk, somewhere beautiful, alone but not lonely.*
+ *Home, after a busy day.*

The ideal configuration of cushions

Life is so often slightly uncomfortable, isn't it? The office chair that doesn't quite support your lower back, the daily commute that requires you to sit or stand awkwardly, time spent waiting in queues or carrying heavy bags ... None of it is painful, but it's not exactly comfortable.

That's what makes lying on your couch with the ideal configuration of cushions so special. If you can get exactly the right cushions in exactly the right places, there is a deep sense of homecoming as your body eases into absolute comfort. Ahh ...

Similar glimmers:
+ *The word "ease".*
+ *The perfect dressing gown, whatever that means to you.*

A midweek, mid-afternoon lie-down

If you should find yourself in the lucky position of being home in the middle of the week, and you happen not to have a meeting, and you feel a little sleepy, you might find your way to a midweek, mid-afternoon lie-down.

Why does it feel so illegal? Who's going to find us? I have no idea ... But the edge of indulgence is part of the fun.

Similar glimmers:
+ *Lying in bed reading on a cold morning.*
+ *A morning bath, with bubbles, and no time limit.*

Bowing out of an event you don't actually need to attend

You may have been raised or encouraged to attend everything you're invited to (the office networking party, that family event with your cousins you haven't seen in years ...). But you don't actually have to go to All The Things if you don't want to. You get to decide, for yourself.

And when you do – when you honour yourself, and the way you feel – well! Look out world.

Similar glimmers:
+ *Nothing to do, nowhere to be.*
+ *Sneaking away from company for a few quiet moments.*

That first delicious chill in the air

It's the air equivalent of a cool drink of water – that first chill in the air that hints at the seasons changing, that the muggy days of summer are on their way out.

Similar glimmers:
+ *Needing to wear a warm sweater for the first time in months.*
+ *No more feeling too hot!*

Beautiful clouds

"Ah! Look at that!" you might say, noticing, as if for the first time, the fact that the sky is filled with shapes that shift across the sky in various shades of white, grey and silver. Watching the clouds shift and drift is one of the cheapest forms of therapy available. It calms your mind, steadies your breathing and reconnects you to a pace of living that is calm and unhurried.

Similar glimmers:
+ *Sunlight slanting through clouds.*
+ *Waking and sleeping with the sun. It doesn't happen often (and perhaps only when camping?) but waking up at sunrise and going to sleep soon after sunset feels like tapping into the earth's natural rhythm.*

Taking your shoes (or bra) off when you get home

Nothing says, "I'm home" like taking your shoes off, or your bra. The instant relief is immense.

Similar glimmers:
+ *Plugging your phone on charge and ignoring it for the night.*
+ *Watching something silly on TV to unwind.*

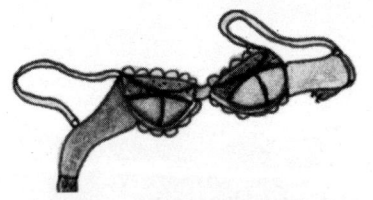
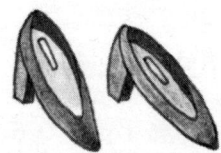

Being early and having some quiet time to chill

I was raised in a chronically late household. It was perfectly normal for us to leave at the last minute, and rush into places just on time or five minutes late. But I recently started experimenting with being early. And I have to tell you: the sense of calm and stillness that results from being early is really special! Does everyone else know this? Everyone else knows this, don't they?

Similar glimmers:
+ *A calm, unhurried pace.*
+ *Feeling organized and on top of things.*

Calming your nervous system

The nervous system is a beautiful thing. While technically it consists of the brain, spinal cord and the body's network of nerves, it is so much greater than the sum of its parts. Calming your nervous system means soothing the sensory signals that are sent between the body and the brain. Go on. Take one conscious breath. The result? You feel more at ease. Life feels simpler.

Similar glimmers:
+ *Sniffing an old book (better yet, an old library or bookstore full of books) or another scent you find soothing.*
+ *Reading a fairy tale: a small portal to wonder.*

An uninterrupted night's sleep

There are so many things that interrupt sleep. Middle-of-the-night worries, unhappy pets, babies and toddlers, the list goes on. An uninterrupted night of sleep is one of the most precious gifts known to mankind. No exaggeration.

Similar glimmers:
+ *Anticipating sleeping in. That sense that you can go to bed whenever you want to because there's nothing to do in the morning.*
+ *An easy commute to work, where everything just flows.*

A perspective-changing walk

You set off on your walk feeling kind of grumpy and weighed down by the world, but somewhere along the way, because of the view (limitless horizons!), or your heart pumping, or because the exercise is releasing endorphins into your system, your perspective shifts. Slightly. And that slight shift is all you need to approach things in a new way.

Similar glimmers:
+ *A micro-nap that shifts your mood.*
+ *A three-minute dance party. One song will do!*

The perfect pillow

Sinking into the perfect pillow is like being greeted with a hug at the end of the day. It's a signal to the nervous system to relax and recharge, and a reminder that sometimes the smaller things in life can have an enormous impact. Don't believe me? Spend a night or two sleeping on a lumpy, flat, saggy pillow and see what it does to your outlook on life!

Similar glimmers:
+ *Lying down in bed after a long day.*
+ *The ideal blanket: not too heavy so you feel like you have a dead weight on you, not too light so you feel a little chilly. The Goldilocks of blankets ... just right.*

A weekend day of no-plans

A few years ago a friend introduced me to the idea of No Plans Sunday, and I could not love it more. It could be a Saturday, if that works better for you – it's less about the day and more about the fact that one whole day on the weekend, you get to do whatever you want to do. No rushing to meet people, running errands or tidying the house because you have guests coming over. You might end up doing any of those things, of course, but it will be by choice and not because your life plan was decided for you weeks in advance.

Similar glimmers:
+ *Unlimited time with your favourite people.*
+ *Choosing not to do anything productive on the weekend. At all. Zero productivity for 48 hours.*

Daydreaming about nothing in particular

Adults are expected to be productive, busy and occupied all the time. Spending time daydreaming – about something that won't and doesn't ever need to happen – feels like a luxury.

Similar glimmers:
+ *Travel daydreams that aren't grounded in reality or budget.*
+ *Pretend house-hunting or imaginary home decor.*

Making homemade pasta

The pleasure that comes from slowing all the way down and making something from scratch, from just three ingredients: eggs, flour and water. And as an added bonus, you can play with the leftover bits of pasta dough, and return to childhood for a few minutes.

Similar glimmers:
+ *Stirring the stock into risotto (a flavourful meditation).*
+ *Cutting shapes out of cookie dough.*

Watching the seasons change

Perhaps, to truly appreciate the changing of the seasons, you need to live somewhere without four distinct seasons. I grew up in Durban, South Africa, where the weather changed from painfully hot and humid to hot, then back to painfully hot and humid. On repeat.

As a result, I truly appreciate watching the seasons change. The way the leaves on the trees go from abundant and green to paler green, yellow, orange and red, and then fall off. It's magical! A visual, visible reminder of the passage of time.

Similar glimmers:
+ *The contrast of orange leaves on blue sky.*
+ *Jumping into a pile of leaves.*

The delicious luxury of a foot massage

There's something about a foot massage that feels very decadent. Someone rubbing your feet, without complaint? How amazing!

Similar glimmers:

✦ *A facial. Layers of scented lotions being rubbed into your skin, one after the other.*
✦ *A soothing yoga class.*

The scent of citrus as you peel an orange

Sometimes all you need to ground yourself in the present moment is a sensory reminder. Your senses pull you to a standstill and say, "Hey! Look at this!" The scent of citrus can do just that.

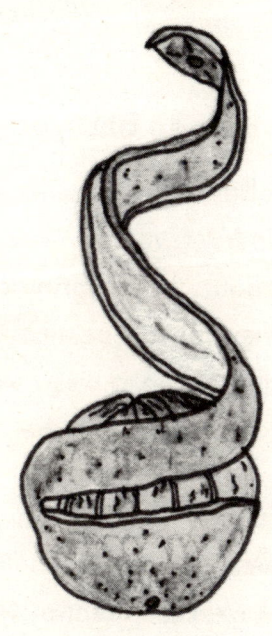

Similar glimmers:

✦ *Cutting into a pepper to find a mini pepper nestled inside.*
✦ *Slicing an avocado that's the perfect ripeness.*

Space and time to think

Things have been so busy! You haven't had a moment to yourself. And then, all of a sudden, the busy dust clears and you find yourself with a small window in which you can pause and think. Inhale, and exhale. Catch your breath.

Similar glimmers:
+ *Time to focus on something that's important to you.*
+ *Quiet time. When my kids were toddlers, I enforced quiet time every afternoon, when they drew or looked at books for an hour, so that I could regain my equilibrium. It's a simple concept but can be so profound: a break to sit quietly and pull yourself together.*

Weather so bad you have to stay indoors

Sometimes the weather is so awful that you have to stay at home. My favourite college professor, Kabi Hartman, used to talk about "the tyranny of the nice day". She felt that when the weather was beautiful and sunny, she was obligated to go out. But when it was cold and rainy, she could stay indoors and read – which is what she wanted to do all along.

Similar glimmers:
+ *Relaxing into a candlelit bubble bath (book optional).*
+ *A weekend getaway with nothing to do but chill.*

Making homemade pesto

Making things from scratch can be so satisfying. This basil pesto is so easy to make, and so tasty. Simply whizz together about 2 cups of fresh basil, ½ cup of olive oil, ⅓ cup of almonds, a pinch of salt, a clove of garlic, ½ cup of grated Parmesan, and you have the easiest-ever pesto-that-goes-with-everything.

Similar glimmers:
+ *Eating your favourite food, often.*
+ *Sitting down to eat a meal quietly and consciously.*

An early night

It's funny how, when you're a kid or a teenager, an early night has no appeal. But as you get older, the lure of an early night beckons. Particularly if you set it up beautifully so your bedroom is the perfect temperature, you're wearing your favourite pyjamas and you have something lovely to read. Mainly, though, an early night is a treat because you know how wonderful you'll feel when you wake up rested tomorrow.

Similar glimmers:
+ *Packing yourself a special lunch for work.*
+ *Making water taste more delicious (ice, lemon, mint ...) so you drink more of it.*

A nap in a hammock

The hammock holds your body like a hug, suspended in mid-air, but totally safe. A light breeze rocks you gently, side-to-side, and you are soothed to sleep. Bliss.

Similar glimmers:
+ *Waking up feeling refreshed from a nap.*
+ *A fresh air break that re-energizes you.*

Crisp morning air

A deep breath of morning air is the most delicious thing: cool and refreshing, like a palate-cleanser to start the day.

Similar glimmers:
+ *The almost imperceptible lightening of darkness into dawn.*
+ *Dozing off in gentle sunshine.*

(Surprise) breakfast in bed

Relaxing in bed, with a coffee and something delicious to eat. And someone who loves you. How wonderful.

Similar glimmers:
+ *A whole day of staying in your most comfortable clothes.*
+ *Returning home after a trip to all your home comforts: your bed, your pillow, your favourite mug.*

Watering the plants

There's a ritualistic aspect to watering the plants at the start or end of the day. Whether you use a little watering can or a hosepipe, if you're watering a few pot plants or a whole garden, it doesn't really matter. Watering the plants is an act that manages to be simultaneously meditative and practical, soothing and essential. How many tasks in life tick all those boxes?

Similar glimmers:

✦ *Unpacking the dishwasher or folding the laundry while listening to your favourite music, and calmly putting everything back where it belongs.*

✦ *Making your bed so Future You has a lovely bed to come home to.*

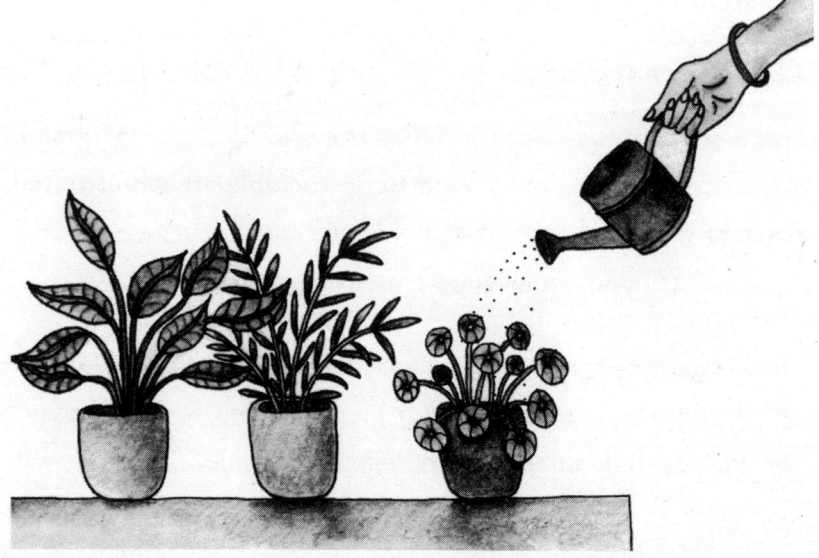

Realizing that your To Do List is never-ending

Perhaps not the most inspiring realization, it's true. But once you recognize your To Do List will never end, you can step away for now and come back to it tomorrow. It'll be okay.

Your To Do List will never be complete. "Complete" is not the goal. The only goal is to do some good work today, and then rest.

Similar glimmers:

+ *Making peace with leaving things unfinished: chores, projects, cups of coffee. Interestingly, leaving some work unfinished for the next day is a productivity hack; it gives you something to finish first thing in the morning and can help you ease into a problem-solving flow the next day.*
+ *Being gentle with yourself.*

4-7-8 breathing

This is such an easy way to reduce the feeling of being frazzled, anxious or overwhelmed. Find a comfortable position to sit in. Breathe in for a count of 4, hold for 7 and breathe out for 8. Repeat until you experience a measure of relief.

Similar glimmers:

+ *Meditating – whatever that means to you.*
+ *Purposefully under-scheduling your life.*

Consciously delaying a big decision

At first glance, this is an odd slice of joy. But it is magical what happens in your subconscious when you consciously delay making a big decision until a specific future date. The key is to specify the future date, and then stop talking or worrying about the decision until that date.

What you'll find is that, like a muddy bucket of water that's been left to rest, the confusion will settle and things will become clear. It's much easier to make a decision once your subconscious has been quietly considering it for a few days or weeks.

Similar glimmers:

✦ *Practising* Memento Mori *(mentioned on page 194) about an issue that's worrying you. Reflect on the worst thing that could happen for two minutes, and then let it go.*

✦ *Going to the cinema to watch a funny movie purely to take your mind off things.*

FINDING JOY ON DARK DAYS

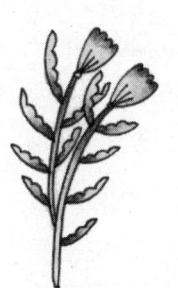
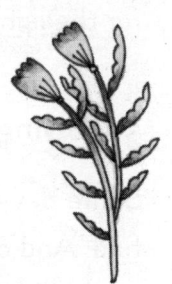

Some days are terrible, horrible, sad or very bad. On those days, it might be even more obvious what your slice of joy is, because nothing else good happened.

But it can also help to take a step back. After my mom died, in the darkest days of my grief, there were times when the only thing I clung to was that the day was over. That I was one day further away from the worst thing that had happened to me, and maybe, hopefully, one day closer to feeling okay again.

On these days, a slice of joy might be making it through today, being able to go to bed or surviving. And that's okay.

✦ Noticing the tiniest glimmers

Sometimes, when I am having a stressful and, frankly, shitty day, the only thing that gets me through it is noticing the glimmers.

It might be some deep breaths of fresh air, noticing pretty flowers or a note of support. If I can notice a glimmer, the day ever-so-slightly brightens. I feel lighter, I can breathe a little deeper and I may have an inkling of a sense of perspective.

This is why slices of joy are so essential. All you need is a sliver for the light to get in, and that sliver can change everything.

✦ Giving joy to others

Some days, I'm not going to lie, glimmers feel impossible to find. And on days like that, I find it helps to offer up a slice of joy to someone else – to reach out beyond yourself and think of what might help others. Again, this can be teeny tiny. Just a few seconds of lightness.

In my constant quest for moments of daily joy, I have found the Magic Banana Message helpful. Using a sharp knife, I write my kids a message on their lunchbox bananas, and it gives me a moment of mirth every morning.

One of my goals in life is to sprinkle our days with a touch of lightness and delight, a few seconds of joy, even on the hard days.

✦ Notice your constant slices of joy

It can be helpful to write down some slices of joy when you're feeling good (or okay), to reflect back on during bad days. These can be things that aren't likely to change: a very comfortable bed, a beautiful view when you look out your window, the perfect mug for that morning cup of coffee … That kind of thing. Can you think of a few now?

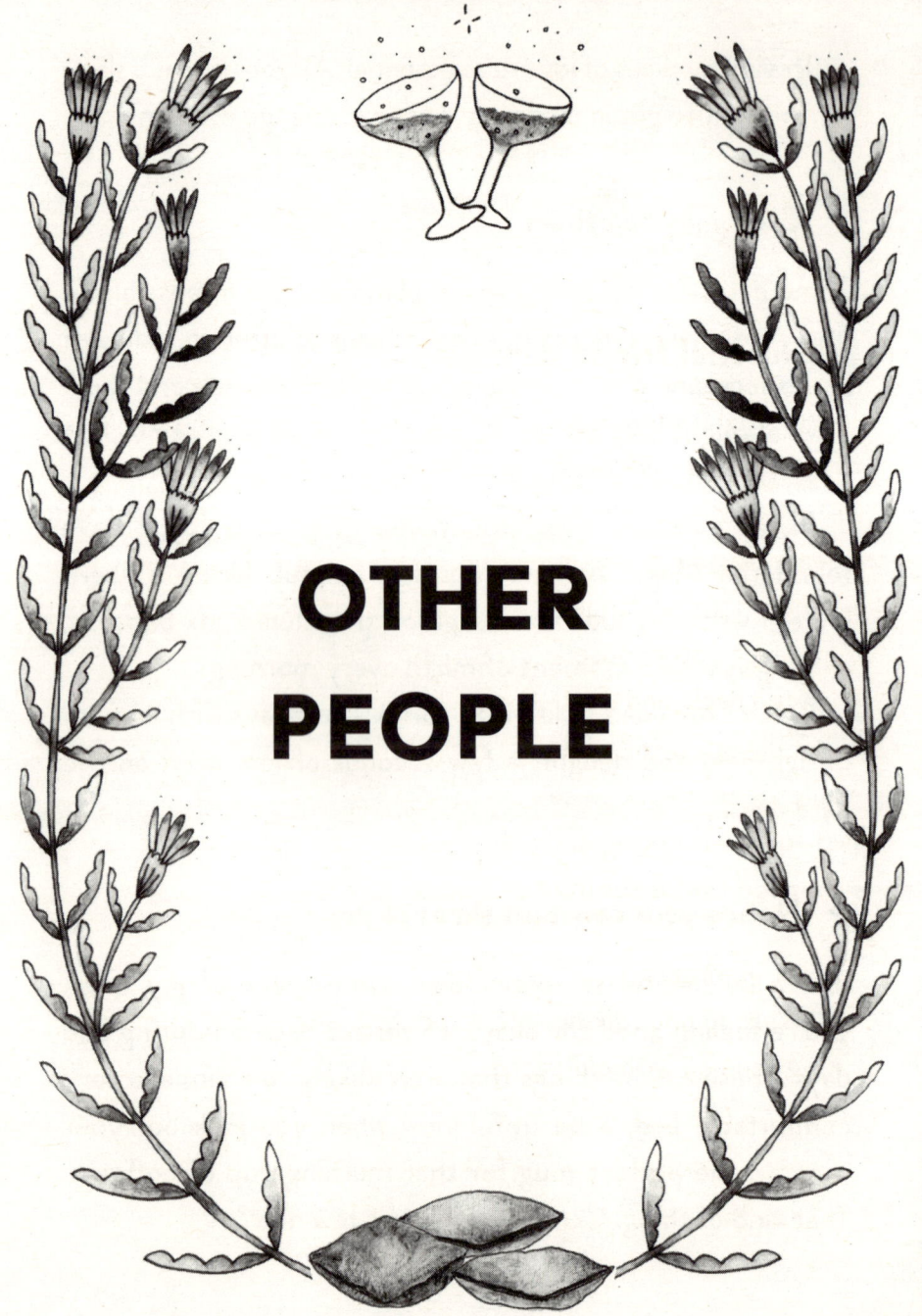

OTHER PEOPLE

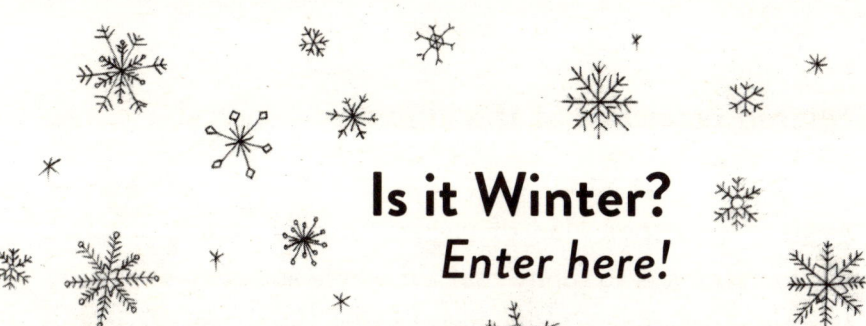

Is it Winter?
Enter here!

Intentional friend date planning

Intentional friend date planning is booking friend dates ahead of time, on a recurring basis. This might seem "too organized", but what it really means is that you get to see your favourite people, regularly, at times that suit both of you. It might be a lunch date, a dance class, a weekly dog walk or a movie. Whatever you choose is up to you. And it's so much better than the back-and-forth scheduling of individual dates, which can take up a lot of headspace. Choosing the people you really, deeply want to see and ensuring you see them often is like future-proofing social connection (and everyone knows how good that is for mental health).

Similar glimmers:
+ *Walking and talking with a special friend.*
+ *A reunion with old friends.*

Shared reactions at the cinema

The movie takes an unexpected turn and the whole cinema gasps ... And then kind of giggles, in mild embarrassment. Or something is so funny that the whole audience can't stop laughing, together. Or you hear sniffles from the row behind you as your own eyes fill with tears.

There are so few truly communal shared moments in life, but that sense of abandon you can get in a cinema during a wonderful movie is one of them.

Similar glimmers:
+ *Being lifted up by a live music performance.*
+ *Hearing someone laugh.*

Being looked after when you're sick

You feel like death warmed-up. All you want is for someone to look after you, serve you exactly the right food and drinks, fluff your pillows, recharge your phone, bring you medicine and just be nice to you.

And then someone does. And while it still sucks to be sick, it now sucks a whole lot less.

Similar glimmers:
+ *Someone laying a blanket over you.*
+ *Holding hands.*

The sibling bond

A whole childhood of shared experiences that you have together. You get it, in a way that other people can't possibly. You understand.

Sibling relationships are wild. You can have the same calves, the same inability to follow directions, the same toenails, and still disagree on profound elements of life. But you'll always have each other – and that has to be worth something.

Similar glimmers:
+ *Dinner with friends, especially old friends.*
+ *An unplugged weekend in nature with friends. There's time to chat and connect. Time to be in nature, stretching your legs. It's the perfect recharge.*

Catching up with a friend in person

You both decide what you want to drink. You settle in, on the couch, round the kitchen table or at the coffee shop. You focus on each other. And you begin. Beautiful. So different to a text or a phone call. So real.

Similar glimmers:
+ *Doing something silly with a friend (jumping over ocean waves, riding a carousel, swinging on swings).*
+ *Scruffy hospitality (not having to tidy up for friends).*

Buying someone something they really want

There are many kinds of gifts. One of my favourites is buying someone something they really want, but for whatever reason (couldn't find it, couldn't afford it) they haven't been able to get. The satisfaction is real!

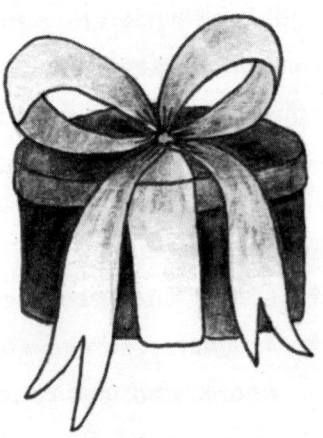

Similar glimmers:
+ *Fulfilling a child's (small, inexpensive) wish.*
+ *Buying fun gifts for someone's birthday (that you know they'll love).*

A small person crawling into your lap

There are times in life when everyone wants to crawl into someone's lap and be comforted. But somehow it's only children who act on that impulse. And when they do, it is one of the sweetest things.

Similar glimmers:
+ *A cute letter written by a young child.*
+ *A cuddle from someone you care about.*

Meeting a friend for lunch on a Monday

Isn't it funny how the day you meet a friend can change the timbre of the interaction? Midweek feels cheeky, somehow, as if putting your work commitments second. A Saturday night feels wilder. A Sunday brunch, lazier.

But Monday! Monday feels downright illegal. I would highly recommend it.

Similar glimmers:
+ *Midweek breakfast with friends: what a slice of joy to start the work day!*
+ *The week between Christmas and New Year, when nobody knows what day it is.*

Seeing a familiar face after a long absence

You haven't seen each other for a few weeks or months, except through screens. And then you see each other in real life and there's a leap of recognition as your gaze lands on their face. An inner sense of: it's you!

Similar glimmers:
+ *Caring about the minutiae in someone else's day ("What did you have for lunch?").*
+ *Coming back to work after a holiday and feeling welcomed into the fold.*

Great service

Service is so often kind of disinterested and lacklustre. So when you get great service from someone it feels special. Something to be noticed, complimented and applauded.

Similar glimmers:
+ *Leaving a great tip for a waiter.*
+ *A phone call to a call centre who really knows what they're doing and resolves your issue quickly, efficiently and politely.*

Meeting a fresh newborn

It's easy to get used to the miracle of life conceptually, but meeting a newborn is a reminder of just how remarkable life is. They are so newly arrived! So only-just-human. This person lived inside another human being until recently. How wild is that?!

Similar glimmers:
+ *Buying adorable things for a new baby.*
+ *Playing peekaboo with a baby for a few seconds.*

A secret smile

You're out in a group and someone says something that you actually cannot believe they uttered out loud. Your eyes widen and you catch the eye of someone who knows you so well they're already smiling a secret smile. You can have a whole conversation within the space of a secret smile. It tells you how known and seen and loved and accepted you are. And how totally whack that comment just was.

Similar glimmers:
+ *A friend or family member knowing exactly how you take your tea or coffee.*
+ *Commiseration: someone knowing how you feel, because the same thing happened to them, and it sucked. There is no need to explain why you feel the way you do. You are just understood.*

Hearing a child laugh

A child's laugh is so purely innocent, delightful and full of wonder. It's like a tinkling bell. Or a magic wish made audible. Listen out for one and you'll see what I mean.

Similar glimmers:
+ *A baby holding tight around your finger.*
+ *Just the right amount of tickle for a true laugh.*

Celebrating with friends

Whatever celebrating means to you: drinks and dancing, a night away, a quiet dinner and soulful conversation, tea and cake. Celebrating is such a vital part of life, and one that's too easy to brush aside. So let's celebrate everything! No excuse is too small for a celebration, as far as I'm concerned.

In fact, one of my reliable adult life hacks is to always have a chilled bottle of bubbly in the fridge. That way, when you get that sense of, "Oh my goodness, I can't believe I've finally finished that project/heard that great news/..." you have a celebration waiting. Just pop the cork!

Similar glimmers:
+ *A road trip with friends – short or long, local or international, big or small group of friends. Doesn't matter! As long as there are tunes, snacks and laughter.*
+ *Dancing: to a great song, played loud, with friends.*

Being offered a piece of someone's snack

You know when you don't want a whole snack, but you still want a taste of whatever it is? That taste is a little slice of joy.

Similar glimmers:
+ *Sharing a pot of tea or coffee.*
+ *Someone helping you clean up a mess you made.*

Crafting with a child

The wild abandon! The mess! The glitter!

Everything I learnt about not saving the good stuff for later (the fancy stickers, the special paper, the fine bone china ...), I learnt from my toddler daughter. She would get art supplies as a gift and use them. Immediately. Completely. Glitter glue pen? Gone in one picture! Fancy expensive stickers? Stuck down on paper, never to be used again.

And why not? I had to ask myself. What am I saving all the good stuff for? This isn't a dress rehearsal, it's the real thing.

Similar glimmers:
+ *Watching kids play in a playground.*
+ *Paddling in the waves with a child.*

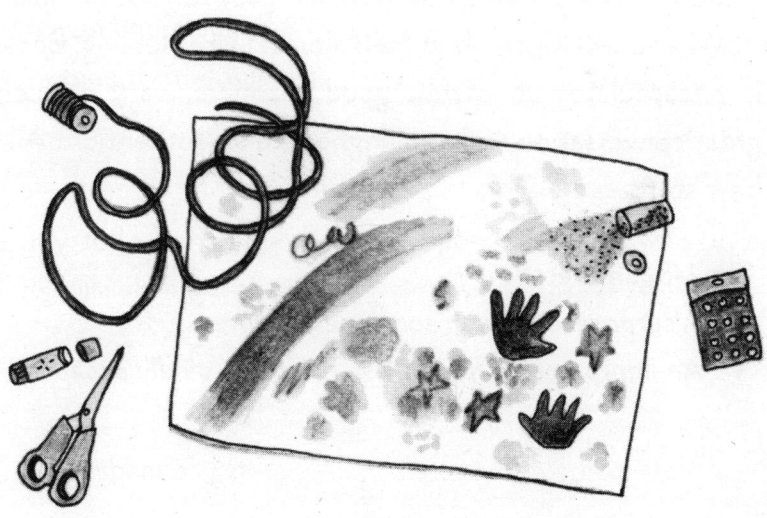

A reciprocal friendship

You know those friendships where it seems like you get as much as you give? You both bring a lot to the relationship, and you both take a lot from it, too. You each have a chance to speak, and to listen. You both leave your interactions feeling filled up.

That's a reciprocal friendship, and if you have one you should thank your lucky stars. They are beautiful.

Similar glimmers:
+ *Being able to answer a call when a friend needs to talk.*
+ *Kindred spirits.*

Good company

Is there a greater compliment than: "They're good company"?

Whenever I bestow it, it feels almost like a blessing. Because it encapsulates so much: good manners, easy ambience, great conversation and a willingness to be authentic ... All the best stuff.

Similar glimmers:
+ *A surprise visit from someone you love.*
+ *An impromptu dinner invite (that you gladly accept).*

Helping a friend reframe an issue

It's about taking a step back and seeing the bigger picture, or looking at things from a different angle. A truly helpful reframe can untangle a sticky situation. It can make you say, "Huh, I never thought of it like that."

It can be tricky to get the clarity necessary to reframe an issue by yourself. Which is why it's so helpful to discuss it with a friend: you can reframe their issues, they can reframe yours, and you both walk away feeling like the world is a kinder, more understandable place.

Similar glimmers:
+ *Venting, uninterrupted, to a friend. And then having that friend gently open a (metaphorical) door so that you can move on from whatever you needed to vent about.*
+ *Sharing knowledge between friends. Life advice, an amazing podcast, the best-ever hand cream, the name of that awesome Mexican place, a helpful financial adviser ...*

"Have a good day!"

Have you noticed this? You pay for your lunch and say, "Have a good day!"

You finish a phone call and say, "Have a good day!"

Almost everyone is walking around like sweet little well-wishers, every day. And sure, maybe you don't mean it too deeply, but it is still a lovely thing to be saying and hearing.

Similar glimmers:
+ *The way the weather is a surprise every year: "It's so cold!"*
+ *Strangers saying, "Bless you!" when someone sneezes*
  – a strange (polite) hangover from the Bubonic Plague.

A lovely schoolteacher

Your paths only cross for a year, but the impact that year makes can last a lifetime. A lovely schoolteacher is one of life's greatest gifts.

Is there a schoolteacher who made a big impact on your life? Take a moment now to remember them. Could you send them an email telling them that? I guarantee that would be a great big slice of joy for your teacher!

Similar glimmers:
+ *An unexpectedly delightful conversation with a stranger.*
+ *Making space for someone in traffic.*

Time with someone you love

It's just the two of you. It might be with a child, a friend, a partner. True one-on-one, undistracted time, is unique enough to be a slice of joy.

Similar glimmers:
+ *Someone you love falling asleep on your lap.*
+ *Doing your favourite thing together (whatever that is).*

Soup for lunch on a winter's day

A bowl of nourishing soup in the middle of a chilly winter's day with a slice of hot, buttered toast is about as good as it gets.

Similar glimmers:
+ *Comfort food for dinner.*
+ *Carpet picnics in front of a fire.*

Putting on clothes warm from the tumble dryer

The hardest part about putting on warm clothes when it's cold outside is stopping the audible "ahhh" of pleasure from escaping your lips when you do.

Similar glimmers:
+ *Wearing a cosy onesie on a frizzling cold day.*
+ *Getting dressed in soft pyjamas and climbing into bed.*

Experiencing magic with a child

I have been lucky enough to experience true magic with my children. One time, a perfectly ordinary tree in our garden sprouted candy canes! Overnight. Another time, my kids planted sweets in a pot of soil and watered them. The next morning, they had grown into lollipops. I know, right? So cool. Impossible to explain
– must be magic.

Similar glimmers:
+ *Hearing a child read for the first time.*
+ *Watching kids hunt for Easter eggs.*

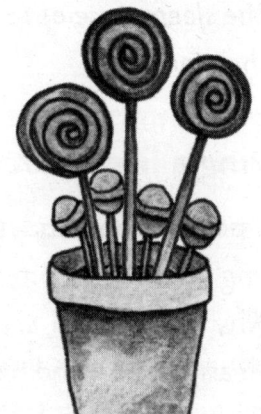

Checking in on a friend

Checking in on a friend is one of the most visible forms of love. It says, "Hey! Life is busy, but I was thinking of you. How are you doing?" It shows your friend that you're thinking of them and have taken the time to reach out. That's love.

Similar glimmers:
+ *A message from a friend.*
+ *"I thought this would make you laugh!"*

Pillow talk

It doesn't really matter what you talk about, it's the cadence of pillow talk that is so sweet. The murmurs, the half-laughs, the sleepy reprimands. Such a joy.

Similar glimmers:
+ *Snuggling when you're half-asleep.*
+ *The sleepy face of someone you love, first thing in the morning.*

Sharing a life-changing moment with a friend

"This podcast/book/quote/idea changed my life." What an opening line! And from there you're off, exploring the topic and why it had such an impact on you and what you could both learn from it and how to make it stick.

Similar glimmers:
+ *Friends who get it.*
+ *Being open to the possibility of your life being changed – even just a little – by another person.*

Pretending you haven't tripped

You're walking down the pavement when you clearly, unmistakably trip over something. And then pretend it didn't happen, even though there are witnesses all around you.

I once saw someone trip over a giant concrete ball as tall as his shin. He caught himself before he fell, spun around spectacularly and carried on walking as if nothing had happened. Why didn't he bow? Everyone would have applauded!

Similar glimmers:
+ *Freudian slips. Particularly if someone tries to cover it up and it is hilariously obvious what their subconscious is trying to say.*
+ *Someone blatantly mispronouncing a word, and sticking by their version no matter what.*

Sitting next to a fire

Whether it's raining or snowing outside, or simply very, very cold, there is such comfort to be gleaned from sitting next to a fire and feeling all toasty warm, when you know you'd be freezing if you stepped outside for even a minute.

Similar glimmers:
+ *Reading in front of the fire on a cold night.*
+ *A heater that brings the room to the perfect temperature.*

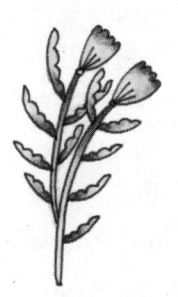

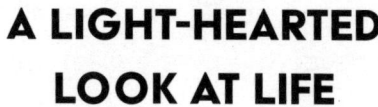
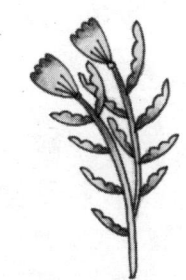

A LIGHT-HEARTED
LOOK AT LIFE

My friend set herself a challenge to find one thing a day that felt fun. Light-hearted. Whimsical. I asked her what kinds of things she discovered, and it was all so achievable:

- ✦ A new red lipstick.
- ✦ Wearing colour instead of black and neutral tones.
- ✦ Small sensory pleasures that felt a little decadent.
- ✦ Not taking herself or her schedule too seriously.
- ✦ The gift of unpredictability: a last-minute dinner date with a friend, a new route home from work, ordering something new for lunch.
- ✦ A little time to herself.

What are three very tiny things you could do to add a light-hearted touch to this week?

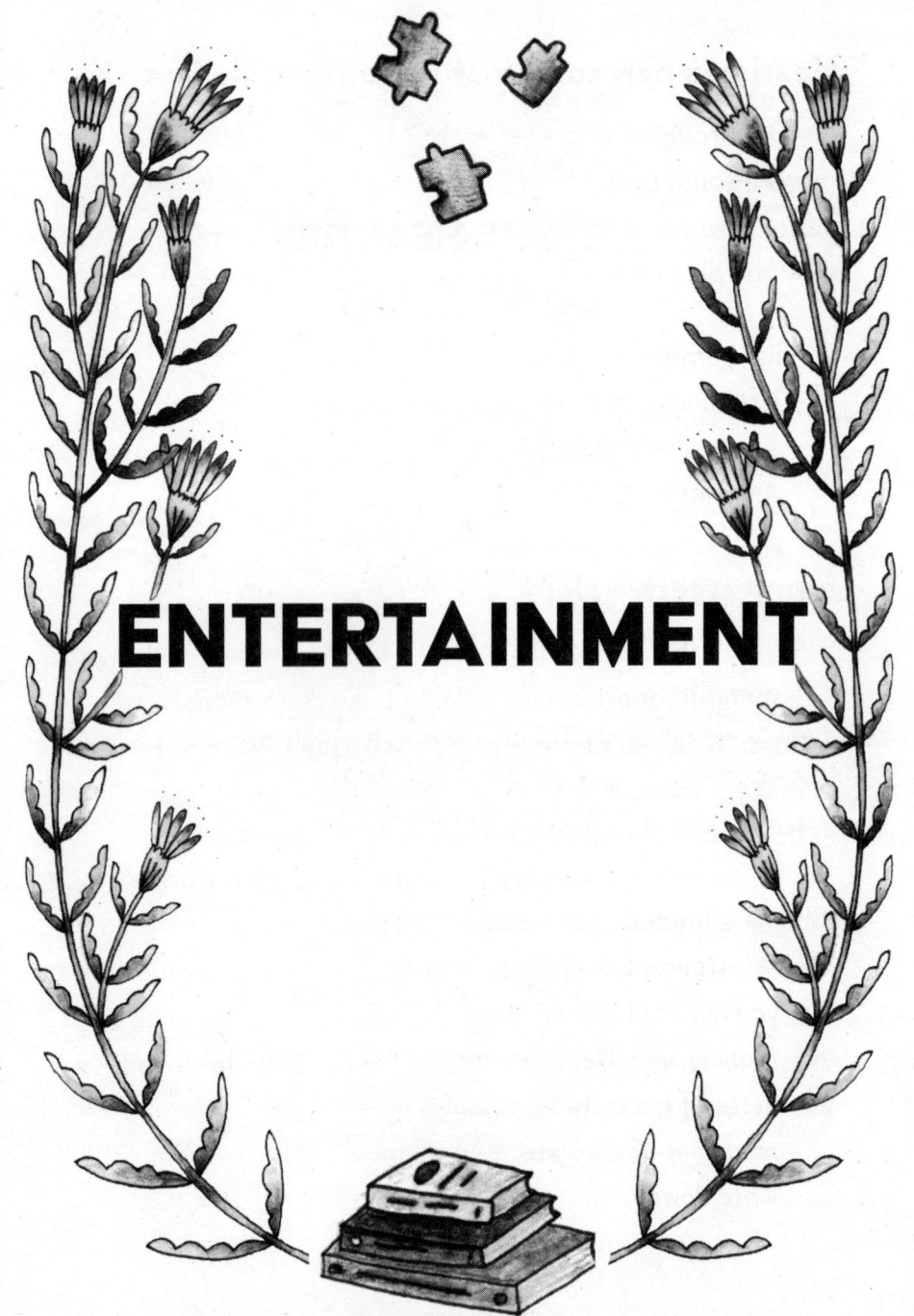

ENTERTAINMENT

Hearing a new song that you absolutely love

I went through a phase when I imagined I had found all the songs I would truly, deeply love. And then I heard something new! I now know that you can be surprised – delighted even – by the passion you feel for a new song.

Similar glimmers:
+ *Listening to exactly what you want to listen to.*
+ *A new album that feels made for you ("I love this song! And this one! And this one!").*

Being creative alongside someone else

Whether the creativity results in anything "good" or "meaningful" doesn't matter, in fact, it's often more fun when it doesn't. What matters is creating alongside one another – making music together, or cooking, painting, drawing or crafting. The shared experience, the mess and the fun.

Similar glimmers:
+ *A restaurant dinner that's so engaging you don't notice you're the last ones there.*
+ *Making something just for the joy of the making. Even better if it's truly transient: a drawing in the sand, a face made out of fruit pieces, or a poem that you don't write down.*

Discussing a good book

It's almost as if you get to experience the pleasure of reading the book twice: once when you're actually reading it, and again when you're discussing it with a like-minded friend.

The characters! The plot twists! Who knows what wonders might be uncovered as you unpack the book together. If you're not a reader, the same can be said of a terrific TV series or movie.

Similar glimmers:
+ *Spending time with a best friend, content in each other's company.*
+ *Rereading a favourite book, and enjoying it just as much.*

Watching a movie that makes you forget yourself

You go into the cinema with the weight of the world on your shoulders. Adulting has ground you down to a husk of your former self. Two hours later, you emerge renewed with a different view on life thanks to the movie you just watched.

Similar glimmers:
+ *Romantic comedies that make you feel good about the world.*
+ *Watching a movie trailer online as a three-minute reward during a busy workday.*

Being outside in freshly fallen snow

Everything has been transformed into mounds of clean, white snow that makes even the most ordinary street look like it's been doused in icing sugar. Yes, the snow will melt and its ugly cousin slush will form. No, this beauty will not last. But while it does … Wow. And you get to walk around in it! Who knew walking could be so entertaining?

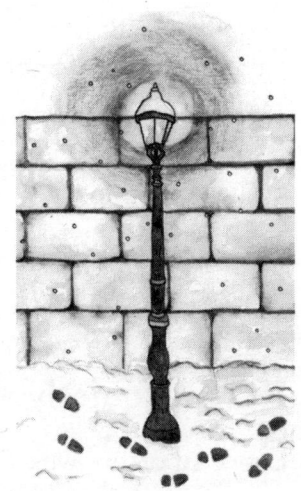

Similar glimmers:
+ *Taking a deep breath of cold winter air, and feeling it travel through your nostrils.*
+ *Burying your nose in a scarf on a chilly walk.*

Finding a meme that speaks to you

There's a particular flavour of surprise and delight that comes from finding a meme that speaks directly to your lived experience. "That's so true!" you think, just for a moment.

Similar glimmers:
+ *Stumbling on unexpected public artworks.*
+ *A clever advert that makes you stop and look.*

Watching an excellent episode of TV

Stories so beautiful, heart-breaking, extraordinary, epic, true and real ... Right here in your home! All that talent and creativity, for your entertainment.

Similar glimmers:
+ *Modern dance that makes your head whirl.*
+ *A truly absorbing play.*

Reading quietly alongside someone you love

Every so often, when I find myself in the midst of a beautiful ordinary moment – like reading quietly alongside someone I love – I'll whisper, "These are the days of our lives."

Nothing is grievously wrong. Nobody is ill. You can afford to live where you live, and eat good food, and you have the space and time to be here, now. Doing this. What abundant good fortune.

Similar glimmers:
+ *Feeling relaxed enough to zone out and gaze at nothing.*
+ *Hanging out with people you love. Just hanging: not doing anything noteworthy that you could report on later. Before every visit, my mom would say to me, "I'm so looking forward to just being together." I think that's one of the highest expressions of love: just being together.*

Hilarious reels

It's difficult to predict what exactly you'll find funny, until it knocks you sideways. But oh my goodness, the glee of that happening is immense! Especially when you've watched the reel 17 times in a row and you're laughing so much that tears stream down your face.

Similar glimmers:
+ *Cat videos. Why are they so funny? Apparently watching cute videos reduces stress and anxiety, but I think it's more to do with the fact that cats are so independent and regal that watching them get flummoxed by simple things is extra surprising and amusing.*
+ *Recipe reels that inspire you to try a new meal.*

Kids listening to a story being read aloud

Maybe it's in your own home or at the local library, or you work in a school. All you have to do is watch a gaggle of children gather around someone reading them a storybook: it's a living testament to the power of story that connects humans one to the other, and a pure positive jolt of energy to behold.

Similar glimmers:
+ *Young kids singing and dancing in unison.*
+ *A poem that makes you understand how you're feeling.*

Poking around in a store to hide from the weather

The weather is unpleasant, there's no getting around it. So, you duck into a store to poke around until the squall passes. But what an unexpected delight! The store is filled with authentically charming things. You get real pleasure from looking around.

Similar glimmers:
+ *Leaving your wet boots at the door and walking around in dry socks.*
+ *Huddling under an awning with total strangers, just until the rain passes.*

Losing yourself in an artwork

You stumble into it almost by chance, walking around looking at all the other artworks. But then this one presents itself and oh! It is just exactly right. Made for you, right here, right now.

Similar glimmers:
+ *Architecture that makes you gasp.*
+ *A photograph that captures life in a way that is almost more real than life itself.*

Finishing a puzzle

You've done the outside, and somehow managed to finish all the sky, and now you're just trying to get this last bit done … And then you see it! The final piece! It all makes sense. The satisfaction is immense.

Similar glimmers:
+ *An excellent board game or game of cards.*
+ *Rediscovering a game you love.*

Making a real effort with your outfit

It might not even be that there's something to dress up for, but some days getting dressed and making a real effort can be such fun. It's elevating getting dressed to a form of entertainment by choosing each element with care.

Similar glimmers:
+ *Treating bedtime as the evening's entertainment. Sometimes you're just Tired with a capital T. On nights like these, I like to treat bedtime as the evening's entertainment. I set everything up for an extraordinary sleep: fresh pyjamas, cup of tea by my bed, hot water bottle waiting. So comforting.*
+ *Turning a night on the couch into something fun: great snacks, dimmed lights, warm blanket, phones out of reach.*

Pop-up books

Don't pretend you don't like them: everyone likes them. The illustrations, the imagination: how do they even *do* that?

Similar glimmers:
+ *Reading an excellent picture book with a child.*
+ *A brilliant graphic novel – so intricate, so nuanced.*

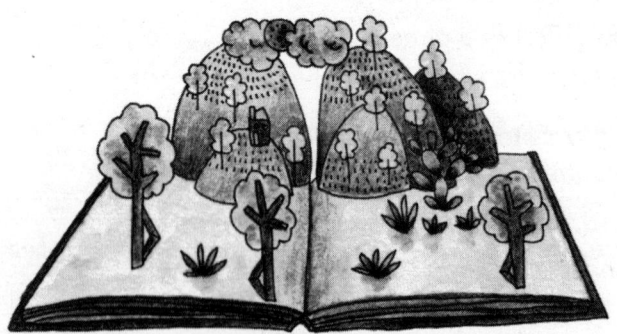

Getting swept up in a classical music performance

You might not fully understand it, but there is something so soaring, sweeping and transcendent about the performance that it carries you along regardless.

Similar glimmers:
+ *A busker who can really play their instrument: literally stopping people in their tracks to listen.*
+ *The band coming back for an encore.*

Listening to a master storyteller

Remember the thrill of being read to as a child? Go and listen to a talented storyteller tell a story! It's mesmerizing how storytellers can use their voices, faces and hands to transform a picture in their head into something you can see vividly. It feels like magic: holding out their hands and saying, "Do you see this thing I created out of thin air?" And you can!

Similar glimmers:
+ *An illusionist who has you authentically befuddled. "How did they do that?"*
+ *Someone getting the lyrics of a song so hilariously, disastrously wrong, and singing them with great abandon anyway.*

Falling in love with a TV character

There are some TV characters that are so real to me I forget they're fictional and that we aren't friends in real life. Have you got one of these? That character who is so funny, or clever, or acts exactly like you wish you could?

Similar glimmers:
+ *The satisfaction of your favourite characters finally getting together.*
+ *The series finale of a beautifully written TV show.*

A podcast so good it makes a commute go quickly

Some commutes seem to crawl past at a glacial pace. Others fly by because you're listening intently to a podcast or interview that is so interesting, unexpected and thought-provoking that your mind is entirely occupied: your neurons firing in all new directions as you start thinking differently about a certain topic.

Similar glimmers:
+ *The music coming through your headphones syncing up so beautifully with what's happening outside that it feels like you've stepped into a movie soundtrack.*
+ *An interview that makes you want to learn more about the person being interviewed.*

Looking forward to your book

You know that book that keeps you turning the pages, and you can't wait to find out what happens next? And all day a part of you is thinking: ooh! I get to go home and read! Blazing through a book because it's unputdownable is a beautiful slice of joy.

Similar glimmers:
+ *An art exhibition that makes you feel all the big feelings.*
+ *The anticipation of a new book by an author you love.*

Savouring a slow-cooked meal

So many of our meals are made on the fly that it feels truly special to savour a slow-cooked meal, one that you know took ages to create. It could be that you enjoyed preparing it slowly, or you deeply appreciate the care and love that went into it.

Similar glimmers:
+ *Leftovers that taste better the next day.*
+ *Going on holiday somewhere there's no signal, so you're forced to read and play board games and chill.*

A snowball fight that leaves you breathless

There are so few occasions to truly let loose as adults. Somehow, wonderfully, snowball fights are still allowed. And there is nothing quite so fun as a snowball fight where you can't breathe properly because you're laughing so hard, and have to call out, "Stop! Stop!" until you catch your breath.

Similar glimmers:
+ *Sledding. Oh my goodness, the thrill of sledding! You're on top of the hill and then whoosh! You're flying!*
+ *The wonder of catching a snowflake (preferably on your tongue).*

Reading until you can't keep your eyes open

The book is so good that you have to keep reading, even though you're so tired your eyes aren't even all the way open any more. And then you drop the book before finally accepting that it's time to go to sleep. Tomorrow is another day!

Similar glimmers:
+ *Stories in front of a fire. Even better if you're curled up under a blanket …*
+ *Reading something (anything!) that makes you snort aloud with laughter.*

Any show that makes you laugh out loud

"Laugh out loud" might be a well-known phrase, but the experience of something being funny enough to actually make you laugh out loud is fairly rare, in my experience. To be funny enough to make you laugh out loud when watching it for the second time is near impossible.

Similar glimmers:
+ *Any show that expands your heart with each episode (for me, Ted Lasso).*
+ *Any show that you have watched so many times that certain references have crept into your daily life without you noticing (for me, Seinfeld).*

A really excellent TED talk

Every so often you'll stumble upon a talk online that is truly meaningful. Fifteen minutes that resonate and teach you something you didn't know. What a joy!

Similar glimmers:
+ *An inspiring quote that connects.*
+ *An excerpt from a book with exactly the wisdom you need for today.*

Rewatching a beloved movie

Logically, the fact that you know exactly what happens and can recite whole lines (whole scenes?) should make it less satisfying to rewatch a movie you love. But somehow, this movie – the one that pushes all your buttons in exactly the right way – is even more satisfying on rewatching. Like eating a meal and knowing you will enjoy every single bite of it.

Similar glimmers:
+ *A movie that helped define your philosophy of life.*
+ *Sharing a favourite movie with your partner, friend or child – and having them love it too.*

Live theatre

The rustle of the audience as they settle into their seats. The lights dimming and actors coming on stage. The vigour and sweat of these talented humans performing live. It's a thrill.

Similar glimmers:
+ *Watching a ballerina dance.*
+ *Watching a really smart comedian perform live.*

Karaoke

Karaoke is one of those times when anything goes, as long as you throw enough enthusiasm at it. It's an acquired taste, and one you only need to indulge in sporadically, so when you do, make sure to dive in wholeheartedly. It doesn't matter if you're rubbish. In fact, that's part of the fun!

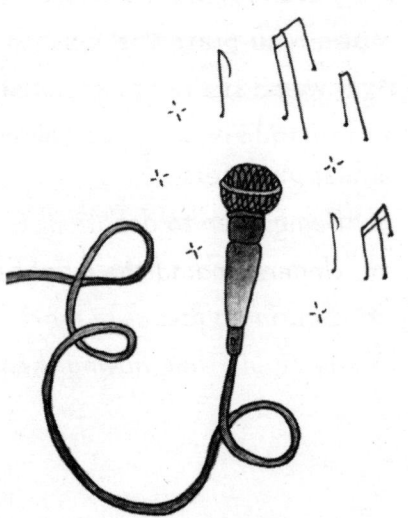

Similar glimmers:
+ *A Murder Mystery party. So ridiculous! So fun.*
+ *Being a tourist in your own city.*

Someone singing to themselves, audibly

I love it when I overhear someone singing to themselves because it seems to me the most obvious example of joy brimming over. There's so much inside it has to come out in song. Even better is when someone is singing to themselves and someone else joins in. That's a double glimmer right there!

Similar glimmers:
+ *Hearing a really excellent whistler belting out a tune.*
+ *Someone quietly humming to themselves without noticing it.*

A thought-provoking documentary

You had a pretty confident worldview on the topic, and then you watched this documentary, and now you're not nearly so sure you grasp the full complexity of the situation, at all. That's good stuff.

Similar glimmers:
+ *Being open to debate about something (anything).*
+ *Understanding the story behind the headlines.*

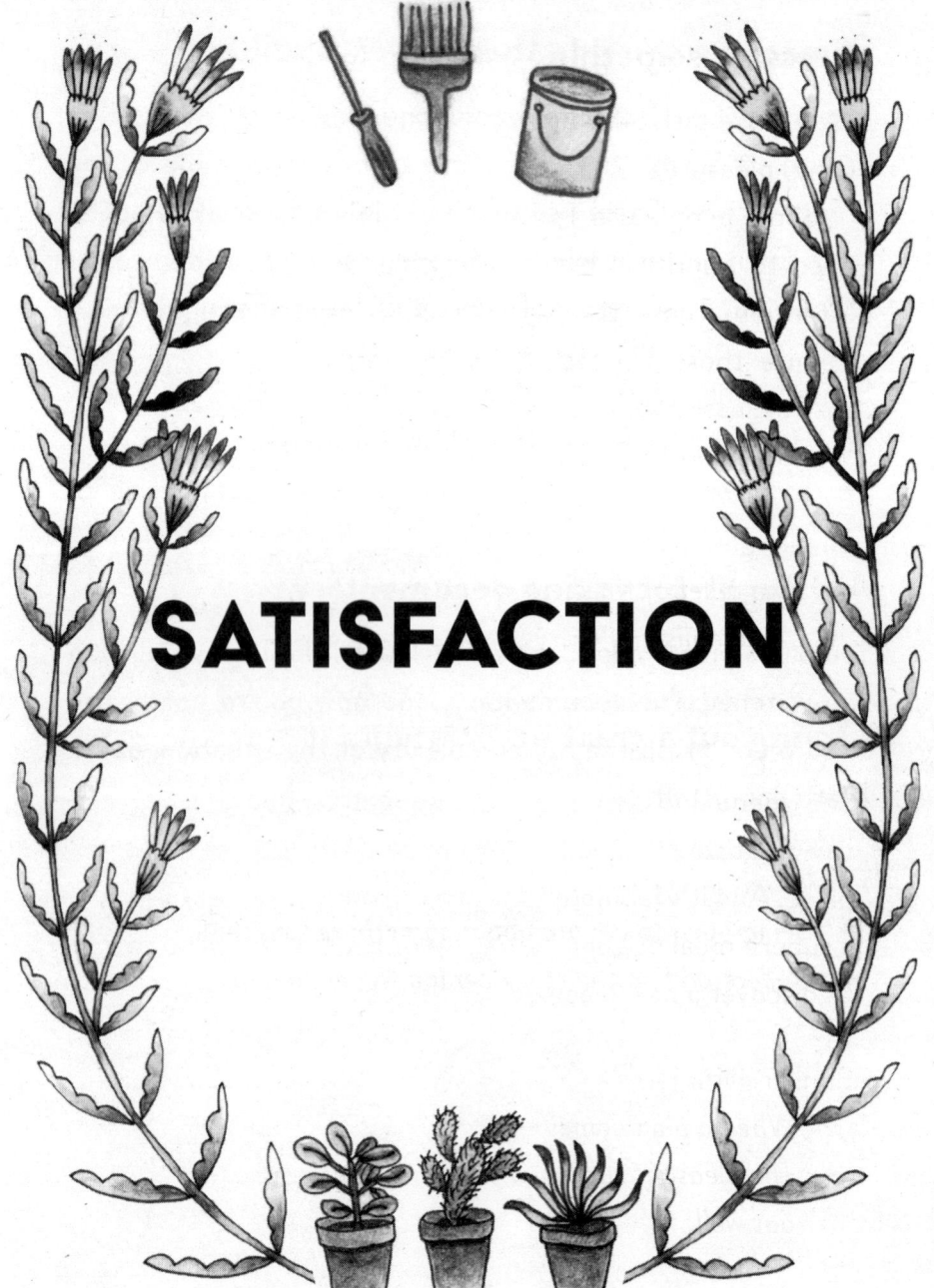

SATISFACTION

Crossing something off your To Do List

Deleting a task off your To Do List is one of adulthood's true (tiny) pleasures.

Some people use To Do Lists as reminders of things they need to prioritize: big, meaty tasks that require significant attention. These take ages to cross off, of course. Others itemize those big tasks into smaller, bite-sized chunks so that at least every day they can cross an item off their list. Whatever works for you!

Similar glimmers:
+ *The relief of finishing a hard task.*
+ *Accomplishing everything you wanted to in a day.*

Trying out a great new restaurant

The menu looks promising, and you've heard some good things, so you decide to take the plunge and try out that new place. And it's fabulous! You get the double endorphin rush of a superb meal out *and* being one of the first people you know to discover a new place. Instant street cred.

Similar glimmers:
+ *When a plan comes together.*
+ *The pleasant surprise of a new dinner recipe that turns out well.*

A dirty windshield made clean

It's muddy, speckly and smeary and then, in a moment, it's sparkling clean. Almost as good as when it's raining heavily and the windshield wipers make an audible "whoosh" as they sluice across the windscreen.

Luckily, these slices of joy don't require owning a car – the sensation is the same whether it's your own car, a taxi or a bus.

Similar glimmers:
+ *Pulling out a patch of weeds, especially after rain.*
+ *Cleaning your glasses – instant better vision!*

A really excellent slice of cake

One day, you are served a really excellent slice of cake, and your perception of what cake can be changes entirely. It turns out it can be exactly the right sweetness, moist but not too moist, the ideal crumb, the perfect marriage between soft cake and creamy icing, with just a hint of freshness to cut through the rich flavour. It is a rapture of cake, a song sung by cake angels and brought to earth for you to eat, right now.

Similar glimmers:
+ *Hot, buttered toast, all oozing and dripping with butter.*
+ *Really fizzy sparkling water.*

Selling something unwanted

It is, in your opinion, a hunk of junk, so you decide to sell it. And someone is so happy, so authentically delighted to buy it from you, and off it goes to its new home.

Similar glimmers:

+ *Resisting the urge to buy anything from a store you like, because you don't actually need anything.*
+ *Finding the right colour paint from all the swatches.*

Sewing on a replacement button

Your shirt is missing a critical button and, therefore, unwearable. It languishes in your wardrobe for days (possibly weeks?). And then, one day, you sew on a replacement button. It takes all of three minutes, from finding the needle to snipping the thread when it's complete. And suddenly your shirt is fixed!

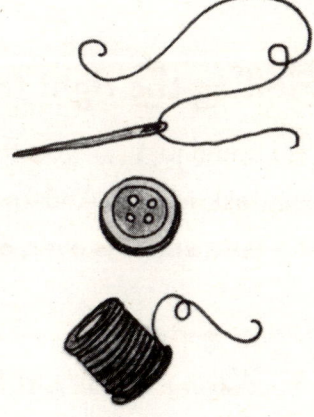

Similar glimmers:

+ *A watering can that pours without dripping.*
+ *Sliding a piece of paper into a plastic sleeve.*

Being "Today Years Old" when you learnt something

I love this phrase: it makes the learning of new information both playful and a thing to aspire to. I've most often seen it used when someone learns a fact or a life hack that they feel they should have known years ago – something that seems obvious to everyone else or is generally accepted as common knowledge.

For example: I was Today Years Old when I learnt that the hole in the pasta spoon is to measure one serving of spaghetti. Huh! You learn something new every day.

Similar glimmers:
+ *Having (all) your questions answered.*
+ *When you teach a child (or pet!) something and they get it first time.*

Finding the right tool for a task

"If I could just ... " you think, trying to figure out how to make this task easier. And then you just find the perfect tool for the task, and it is over, done, completed within minutes. Yay!

Similar glimmers:
+ *Waking up early without an alarm.*
+ *A can opener that works first time.*

The exact right word

Whether in a word game or in conversation, or when writing something, it's a particular pleasure when the precise word you've been excavating for unearths itself like a rare gem.

Similar glimmers:
+ *Finding a "like new" copy of an out-of-print book.*
+ *Being right on time.*

Finishing a jar of something

It is done. You have scraped out the last possible vestige and now all that is left is a satisfyingly empty jar. Well done, you.

Similar glimmers:
+ *The satisfying crunch of slicing through a pile of spinach. Or chopping a crunchy apple.*
+ *Finally reading that book or article you've been meaning to.*

Finding the perfect plant for a pot

Like successfully matchmaking a couple, pairing a plant and a pot is a gift that keeps on giving, every time you look at it.

Similar glimmers:
+ *A house plant that thrives on neglect.*
+ *Eating something you grew yourself.*

Meeting a goal (no matter how small)

Did you ever have a reward chart when you were a child? I often think adults need them. For all the daily drudge you don't enjoy but have to do anyway. You could get a little star for every day you exercised in the cold, or went to work instead of huddling under the covers, or paid your bills on time. And then a prize at the end of the month! (Hang on, maybe that's what payday is?)

Meeting any goal, no matter how small, is worthy of reward. What tiny goal could you achieve this week?

Similar glimmers:
+ *A tidy bookshelf: all the books in an order that makes sense to you.*
+ *The first spray of perfume from a new bottle.*

A small DIY project, successfully completed

Something was broken that needed to be fixed. Or something needed new life breathed into it, and you did it! It may only have been a small DIY project, but the impact it makes on daily life is big (well, big enough to celebrate).

Similar glimmers:
+ *Oiling a squeaky door.*
+ *Erasing a whiteboard so it's totally clean.*

Kneading dough

There's no better way to vent frustration or unwind after a busy day than kneading dough. The gentle rhythm, the need for contained strength, the enforced slowing down, the necessity of time to do what needs to be done before you can be finished ... It's a very practical meditation.

Similar glimmers:
+ *Mixing batter by hand.*
+ *Baking a cake successfully (the relief of it coming out of the tin never gets old!).*

Being bad at a new thing but enjoying it anyway

I'm not sure why, but it seems as if an unwritten code of adulting is expecting to be good at all things as soon as you try them. Which is blatantly impossible, of course, and something that I would never lead a child to believe, but is something that I somehow swallow whole?

So, it is refreshing to attempt something new and be truly awful at it, but still enjoy the experience.

Similar glimmers:
+ *Being taught the basics of a topic you care about and want to understand better.*
+ *A risk that paid off.*

A beautiful cheese board

If they conceived of a test to show that you're a real adult, I would argue that a beautifully put together cheese board should be it. It's a work of art in edible form: different cheeses, some grapes and fresh figs, the ideal amount of preserves and an elegant array of biscuits and breads and other nibbles.

Similar glimmers:
+ *Reviving a dying fire.*
+ *Stumbling on a secret spot in a busy public park.*

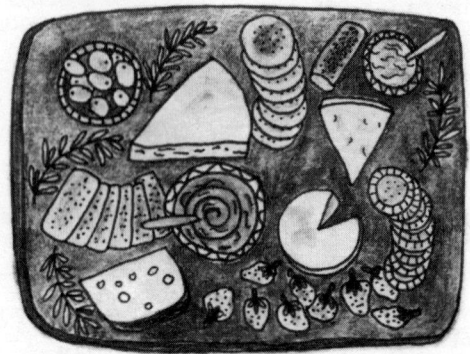

A good hair day

A good hair day can delight you every time you look in the mirror.

Similar glimmers:
+ *Fresh nails after a chipped manicure or pedicure.*
+ *Combing easily through usually-knotty hair.*

A square of chocolate dipped into a hot drink

You may not have experienced this particular joy, so allow me to outline the method:

1. First, make yourself a cup of tea or coffee.
2. Then, break off a square or two of chocolate.
3. Now, dip one end of the chocolate into your drink, just long enough to melt the end a little.
4. Nibble the melty end off. And repeat.

You can thank me later, once you've washed the melted chocolate off your hands.

Similar glimmers:
+ *A cup of hot chocolate on an icy day.*
+ *A glass of red wine in front of a fire.*

Parallel parking in one try

You glide into the space perfectly, just the right distance from the kerb and the cars around you. That feels like an action to be applauded, any time it happens.

Similar glimmers:
+ *Biting into a chocolate bar.*
+ *A train arriving exactly on time.*

Eating exactly what you feel like

You're hungry. You know precisely what you feel like eating. And then? Most of the time you eat something else, because you can't get exactly what you want. But sometimes you can!

Similar glimmers:
+ *A beautifully laid tea party table.*
+ *Throwing a piece of paper into the bin from a distance – and getting it in.*

Popping bubble wrap

You don't have to be a kid to enjoy popping bubble wrap – you just have to be human.

Similar glimmers:
+ *Squeezing out the first bit of a new tube of toothpaste.*
+ *Icing a cake on a turntable.*

Noise-cancelling headphones

Being able to block out noises from people, stores and – my worst – airports has changed my life. Pockets of calm.

Similar glimmers:
+ *Plentiful tissues when you need them.*
+ *Finding unexpected money in a bag or jacket pocket.*

Finding a lost sock

You are just on the verge of relegating the single sock to the recycling, when its partner is found! And order is restored in the world.

Similar glimmers:
+ *Something lost is found.*
+ *Finding the right type of batteries in the drawer.*

Doing a pee when you've been holding it in

The relief of this feeling is exactly commensurate to how desperately you need to pee. Just a little urgency? Just a little relief. Can't think of anything except your exploding bladder? Immense and powerful relief.

Similar glimmers:
+ *Eating when you're starving hungry.*
+ *Putting on socks when your feet are freezing.*

Striking a match and having it light immediately

It can be that small, and that satisfying.

Similar glimmers:
+ *The toaster popping up a perfectly toasted slice of bread.*
+ *Catching a falling object before it lands on the floor.*

Starting a log fire from scratch

There's no hope. There's no hope. There's maybe a teeny little bit of hope? There's hope! It's catching! It's catching! It's blazing. Wow!

Similar glimmers:
+ *"Please send me the recipe?" They do. And it's easy!*
+ *Sweeping up loose ends: the final details of a project, the last spell-check of a document, packing the stray things before leaving home. That sense of "it's nearly done, let me just tidy up this final bit".*

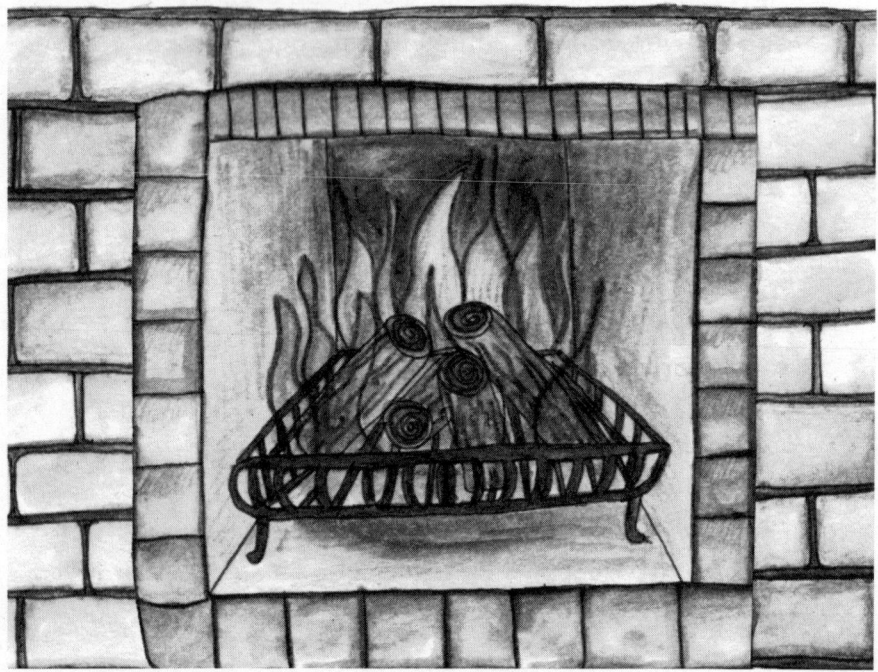

A speedy response to an email

You send off an important email and start telling yourself the story of how long you can reasonably expect to wait before getting impatient for a response. But before you even get to the end of the story, the person has replied! What joy! What luck!

Similar glimmers:
+ *Finding a book you've been wanting to read at the library.*
+ *Someone connecting you to the right person.*

Figuring out how to do something

You've never done it before. You don't know how to do it or who to ask for help. So you have to figure it out with a combination of online videos, sheer dogged determination and just having a go. And then you do it! What a rush.

Similar glimmers:
+ *Completing a creative project to the best of your ability.*
+ *An early start to the day because you're so excited to begin working on something.*

Voicing a new idea eloquently

If you're like me, every so often you'll come across a new idea that excites you, and desperately want to share it with someone in particular. But when it comes time to explain what makes it so exciting and why you think they would really care, words just don't come. So, on the odd occasion that an idea sparks your interest and you are able to share it eloquently, well! That is cause for celebration.

Similar glimmers:
+ *Mastering a new skill. You had no idea how to do it, and now it's in your toolbox of skills! Look at you.*
+ *A productive hour doing what you love most.*

Reflecting on the day's slices of joy

The day has come to an end. Like every day, there have been some good bits and some challenging/boring/uncomfortable parts. But you're not doing an hour-by-hour analysis. All you're doing is looking for one or two slices of joy from your day, a moment or two of brightness amid the blah. A couple of tiny glimmers.

Similar glimmers:
+ *Gratitude for small blessings.*
+ *This moment, right here.*

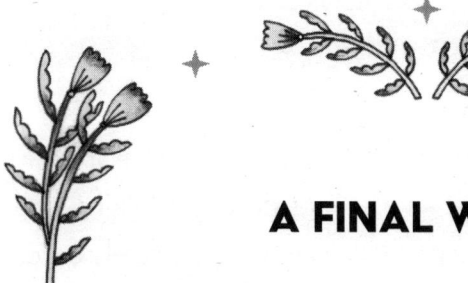
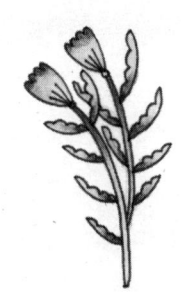

A FINAL WORD

It will come as no surprise that there are more than 365 glimmers to be found in daily life. It's a never-ending list. In fact, just this morning I realized I'd found another: when you dip a toast soldier into a soft-boiled egg and the yolk overflows down the side like lava from a volcano. So satisfying!

Also, origami cranes! How did I forget origami cranes? I fold them constantly, as a tiny little meditation for my hands, and gift them on strings for baby showers and weddings. Also, pass-the-parcel! That should be on the list. And the calm trance of staring out a window at scenery rolling past on a road trip. The satisfaction of burning a candle all the way to the end. I could go on, and on, and on.

But that's not the point. It's not just my joy journey, is it? It's yours now. I leave you with the tools that helped pick me up out of a funk (over and over again) and into a lighter way of being in the world. I hope they can help you too.

Let's walk forward, together. Into a future that is unknown and no doubt challenging, but that is also – always and forever – glimmering with slices of joy. No matter what.

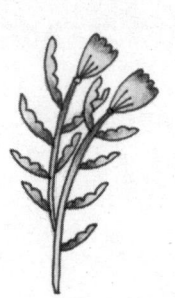

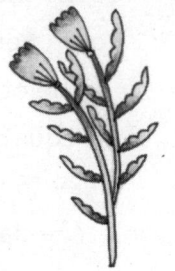

ACKNOWLEDGEMENTS

Writing a book is such a funny thing because half of it is sitting alone doodling on a document, and the other half involves a whole (magical!) team of people bringing that document to life.

This book wouldn't have been possible without my delightful agent Kay Peddle, from Colwill & Peddle, who patiently listened to so many long voice notes as I figured out exactly what this book should be.

I was lucky enough to work with a dream team at Watkins Publishing: my lovely editor Sophie Blackman, alongside Brittany Willis, Gigi St John, Sneha Alexander and Hayley Moss. Thank you for all your help and enthusiasm! Becky Alexander swooped in to do a "light edit" and made *Daily Glimmers* so much better with her eagle eye – thank you for your thoughtful suggestions.

And then, of course, there's Lauren Fowler and her beautiful illustrations, which I insisted on not only in this book but in my previous book, *The Grief Handbook*, and which adorn the walls of my home and office. Thank you for doing your (wonderful) thing once again!

The other half of writing a book – doodling on a document – requires a surprising amount of support, which I was so lucky to have from all sides.

My dad Raymo and brothers Bongin, Smile and Mouldy, are a constant presence. My dearest Kindle Club, Becks and Mieks, kept me going with encouragement and our never-ending Kindle Club train of voice notes (choo-choo!).

Jessy remains my cheerleader and best-ever first reader – thank you, my kindred spirit.

Squirrel is always there, thank heavens. Cath walked beside me, as she always does, and Debbie guided me through the dark days.

And then, of course, there are my favourite people in the entire world – beloved Marky, Arty and Ella. Thank you for giving me the space to write this book, even though it took so much longer than you thought ("You're *still* writing your book, Mom?").

You are my daily glimmers.

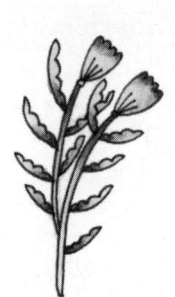

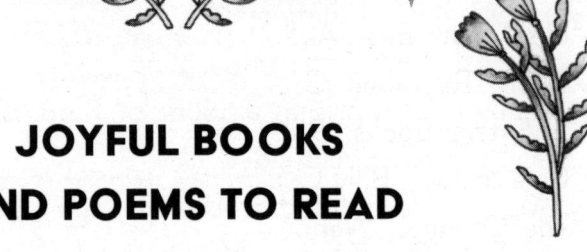

JOYFUL BOOKS
AND POEMS TO READ

Books

The Book of Joy, His Holiness the Dalai Lama and Archbishop Desmond Tutu with Douglas Abrams, Random House USA Inc, 2016

The Book of Delights, Ross Gay, Coronet, 2020

The Little Book of Joy, Joanna Gray, Quadrille Publishing Ltd, 2022

The Daily Stoic, Ryan Holiday and Stephen Hanselman, Profile Books, 2016

A Guide to the Good Life, William B. Irvine, Oxford University Press Inc, 2009

The Joy of Small Things, Hannah Jane Parkinson, Guardian Faber Publishing, 2021

Poems

"Idea", Kate Baer, *And Yet*, Harper, 2022

"Rain", Raymond Carver, *All of Us: The Collected Poems*, Vintage Books, 1996

"Ode to Joy", Billy Collins, *The Atlantic*, November 2021

"The Orange", Wendy Cope, *The Orange and other poems*, Faber & Faber, 2023

"i thank You God for most this amazing", E. E. Cummings, *Xaipe*, Oxford University Press, 1950

"The Cure For It All", Julia Fehrenbacher, *Poetry of Presence: An Anthology of Mindfulness Poems*, Grayson Books, 2017

"Coconut", Paul Hostovsky, *Bird in the Hand*, Grayson Books, 2006

"Warning", Jenny Joseph, *The Listener*, 1961

"Small Kindnesses", Danusha Laméris, *Bonfire Opera*, University of Pittsburgh Press, 2020

"Don't Hesitate", Mary Oliver, *Devotions: the selected poems of Mary Oliver*, Penguin Press, 2017

"So Much Happiness", Naomi Shihab Nye, *Words Under the Words: Selected Poems*, Far Corner Books, 1995

"Good Bones", Maggie Smith, *Good Bones*, Tupelo Press, 2017

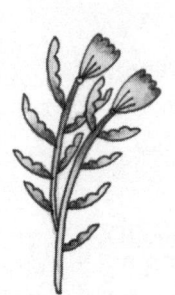

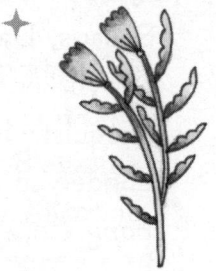

REFERENCES

1 Dana, Deb, "On Glimmers", *Rhythm of Regulation*, rhythmofregulation.com/glimmers

2 Marie, Helen, @h.e.l.e.n.m.a.r.i.e on Instagram, 12 April 2023, instagram.com/p/Cq7OgDGoW3_/

3 Tan, Chade-Meng, *Joy on Demand: The Art of Discovering the Happiness Within with Chade Meng Tan at HAP20*, YouTube, 27 August 2021, youtube.com/watch?v=H5mXW_VXanE

4 Keltner, Dacher, "The Thrilling New Science of Awe", *On Being with Krista Tippett*, 2 February 2023, onbeing.org/programs/dacher-keltner-the-thrilling-new-science-of-awe/

5 University of Sussex, "It's true: The sound of nature helps us relax", *ScienceDaily*, 30 March 2017, sciencedaily.com/releases/2017/03/170330132354.htm

6 University of Sussex, "It's true: The sound of nature helps us relax", *ScienceDaily*, 30 March 2017, sciencedaily.com/releases/2017/03/170330132354.htm

7 Sedaris, David, "Pearls", *The New Yorker*, 10 May 2021, newyorker.com/magazine/2021/05/17/pearls

8 Niequist, Shauna, *I Guess I Haven't Learned That Yet*, Zondervan, April 2022

9 Fong Yan, A., Cobley, S., Chan, C. et al., "Dancing may be better than other exercise for improving mental health", The University of Sydney, 12 February 2024, sydney.edu.au/news-opinion/news/2024/02/12/dancing-may-be-better-than-other-exercise-for-improving-mental-h.html

10 Heyes, Cressida, "Sleep is the New Sex", *ERA*, 11 October 2016, era.library.ualberta.ca/items/328dabdc-8526-4bf2-9fb0-b112a0c825f4

11 *APA Dictionary of Psychology*, "Joy", dictionary.apa.org/joy

12 Ricard, Matthieu, "The habits of happiness", YouTube, 15 April 2008, youtube.com/watch?v=vbLEf4HR74E&t=6s

13 Lambert, Craig, "The Science of Happiness", *Harvard Magazine*, January–February 2007, harvardmagazine.com/2007/01/the-science-of-happiness-html

14 Murphy, Carrie, "This Is How Joy Affects Your Body", *Healthline*, 22 August 2018, healthline.com/health/affects-of-joy

15 Suttie, Emma, "Feeding Your Heart and Soul with Joy", *The Epoch Times*, 4 March 2022, theepochtimes.com/health/feeding-your-heart-and-soul-with-joy-4305701

16 Schaffner, Anna Katharina, Ph.D, "Hedonic vs. Eudaimonic Wellbeing: How to Reach Happiness", *Positive Pyschology*, 6 March 2023, positivepsychology. com/hedonic-vs-eudaimonic-wellbeing/

17 Ratcliffe, Susan, *Oxford Essential Quotations (4 ed.)*, Oxford University Press, 2016

18 Woolf, Virginia, *The Common Reader*, Harcourt, Brace & Company, 1925

19 Woolf, Virginia, *To the Lighthouse*, The Hogarth Press, 1927

20 The 5 Love Languages, 5lovelanguages.com

21 *Collins Dictionary*

22 Shaw, Keeley, @keeleyshawart on Instagram, 14 November 2022, instagram.com/p/Ck9auSlJg_L/

23 Time to Think, timetothink.com

24 King's College London, "Exposure to trees, the sky and birdsong in cities beneficial for mental wellbeing", *ScienceDaily*, 9 January 2018, sciencedaily.com/ releases/2018/01/180109214943.htm

25 Burnout, burnoutbook.net

26 Gay, Ross, "On the Insistence of Joy", *On Being with Krista Tippett*, 25 July 2019, onbeing.org/programs/ross-gay-on-the-insistence-of-joy/

27 Irvine, William B., williambirvine.com/

28 Ahmed, Sara, *The Promise of Happiness*, Duke University Press, April 2010

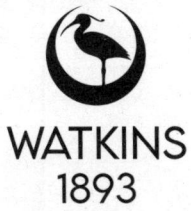

WATKINS
1893

The story of Watkins began in 1893, when scholar of esotericism John Watkins founded our bookshop, inspired by the lament of his friend and teacher Madame Blavatsky that there was nowhere in London to buy books on mysticism, occultism or metaphysics. That moment marked the birth of Watkins, soon to become the publisher of many of the leading lights of spiritual literature, including Carl Jung, Rudolf Steiner, Alice Bailey and Chögyam Trungpa.

Today, the passion at Watkins Publishing for vigorous questioning is still resolute. Our stimulating and groundbreaking list ranges from ancient traditions and complementary medicine to the latest ideas about personal development, holistic wellbeing and consciousness exploration. We remain at the cutting edge, committed to publishing books that change lives.

DISCOVER MORE AT:
www.watkinspublishing.com

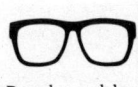

Read our blog

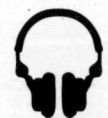

Watch and listen to
our authors in action

Sign up to
our mailing list

We celebrate conscious, passionate, wise and happy living.
Be part of that community by visiting

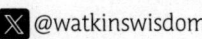 /watkinspublishing   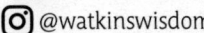 @watkinswisdom
/watkinsbooks   @watkinswisdom